"This is a rare gem of a book that is engaging, interesting, and instructive to people at all levels of knowledge about schizophrenia. Everyone ranging from established researchers to seasoned clinicians to family members to consumers with lived experience to those with a passing interest in schizophrenia will learn something new and valuable from this engrossing and authoritative book written by a team of experts in the field."

Kim T. Mueser, PhD, *Professor, Center for Psychiatric Rehabilitation, Boston University, USA*

"For the average person, schizophrenia remains shrouded in mystery. This practical book explains what it is in everyday language and shows how so much can now be done to help the sufferer return to a normal life."

Sir Robin Murray, FRS, *Professor of Psychiatric Research, Institute of Psychiatry, King's College, London, UK*

"This is a comprehensive and accessible, up to date summary of what we know and need to know about schizophrenia. I highly recommend this book for clinicians, family members and peers who live with the condition."

Ken Duckworth, MD, *Chief Medical Officer, National Alliance on Mental Illness (NAMI), Author of* You Are Not Alone, *NAMI's bestselling book, USA*

"It is incredibly rare to find a book about schizophrenia that is both scientifically accurate and at the same time accessible to readers in the community as well as clinicians and researchers. Having a common base of understanding about schizophrenia provides a valuable tool for enhancing services and care for the many patients and families who face its challenges."

Nina R. Schooler, *Professor of Psychiatry and Behavioral Sciences, State University of NY Downstate Health Science Center, USA*

Schizophrenia

This second edition of *Schizophrenia: A Practical Primer*, includes decades of clinical and research experience in the field and helps readers understand what schizophrenia is and how it is managed.

Schizophrenia is a devastating illness that affects more than 50 million people worldwide. Written to help anyone who is faced with managing schizophrenia, whether as a clinician, patient, friend, or family member, this accessible book is an ideal first stop for practical, up-to-date information. It includes an overview of schizophrenia and provides answers to common questions that arise on different aspects of the illness, such as: diagnosis, pharmacological and psychotherapeutic management, treatment challenges and achieving recovery. Beyond these key issues, the book includes developments in the neurobiology of the illness, foreseeable developments and the history of schizophrenia. It also includes brief, realistic case vignettes adapted from clinical experience, and questions interspersed throughout the book to aid understanding.

This book is essential for professional trainee and early-career mental-health workers, such as psychiatrists, psychologists, social workers, counselors and nurses, and is written to cover in a concise and accessible way what is of immediate and practical relevance to gain familiarity with schizophrenia.

Matcheri S. Keshavan, MD, is Stanley R Cobb Professor and Academic Head of Psychiatry, Beth Israel Deaconess Medical Center and Massachusetts Mental Health Center (MMHC); Harvard Medical School. He has an active clinical practice at the Aspire clinic, BIDMC.

Vinod H. Srihari, MD, is Professor of Psychiatry, and Director of the Program for Specialized Treatment Early in Psychosis (STEP) at the Connecticut Mental Health Center (CMHC); Yale University School of Medicine.

Ravinder Reddy, MD, is former Health Sciences Professor, Department of Psychiatry, University of California, San Diego, School of Medicine; former Psychiatry Training Director at the University of Pittsburgh School of Medicine.

Schizophrenia

A Practical Primer

Second Edition

Matcheri S. Keshavan, Vinod H. Srihari and
Ravinder Reddy

Routledge
Taylor & Francis Group
NEW YORK AND LONDON

Designed cover image: Daniil Peshkov © Dreamstime.com

Second edition published 2024
by Routledge
605 Third Avenue, New York, NY 10158

and by Routledge
4 Park Square, Milton Park, Abingdon, Oxon, OX14 4RN

Routledge is an imprint of the Taylor & Francis Group, an informa business

© 2024 Taylor & Francis

The right of Matcheri S. Keshavan, Vinod H. Srihari, and Ravinder Reddy to be identified as authors of this work has been asserted in accordance with sections 77 and 78 of the Copyright, Designs and Patents Act 1988.

First edition published by CRC Press 2006

Library of Congress Cataloging-in-Publication Data
Names: Keshavan, Matcheri S., 1953– author. | Srihari, Vinod H., author. | Reddy, Ravinder, author.
Title: Schizophrenia : a practical primer / Matcheri S. Keshavan, Vinod H. Srihari, and Ravinder Reddy.
Description: Second edition. | New York, NY : Routledge, 2024. | Includes bibliographical references and index.
Identifiers: LCCN 2023040172 (print) | LCCN 2023040173 (ebook) | ISBN 9781498754798 (pbk) | ISBN 9780367698379 (hbk) | ISBN 9781315152806 (ebk)
Subjects: LCSH: Schizophrenia—Popular works. | Schizophrenia—Popular works.
Classification: LCC RC514 .R3858 2024 (print) | LCC RC514 (ebook) | DDC 616.89/8—dc23/eng/20231107
LC record available at https://lccn.loc.gov/2023040172
LC ebook record available at https://lccn.loc.gov/2023040173

ISBN: 978-0-367-69837-9 (hbk)
ISBN: 978-1-498-75479-8 (pbk)
ISBN: 978-1-315-15280-6 (ebk)

DOI: 10.4324/9781315152806

Typeset in Stone Serif
by Apex CoVantage, LLC

We dedicate this book to the many patients and their relatives who helped us become better clinicians, to our students who helped us become better teachers, to our parents who helped us become better persons and to our wives and children for their unstinting support and encouragement.

Matcheri S. Keshavan, Vinod H. Srihari and Ravinder Reddy

Contents

Preface   xi

1   What is and is not schizophrenia?   1

2   Assessment of schizophrenia   9

3   Social determinants of health affecting assessment   25

4   Schizophrenia, spirituality and religion   33

5   Putting together the (clinical) pieces   37

6   Talking to patients and families   47

7   Early intervention and prevention for schizophrenia   59

8   Managing symptoms and preventing relapse:
     Pharmacological approach   65

9   Psychosocial approaches to improve symptoms
     and functional outcomes   77

10   Managing treatment-related complications   91

11   Suboptimal treatment response   99

12   Medication nonadherence   109

13   Managing decompensation and relapse   121

14   Suicide and violence   129

15   Achieving recovery   135

16   History of schizophrenia   143

17   Who gets schizophrenia and why?   149

18 Neurobiology of schizophrenia   157
19 What does the future hold?   167

Glossary of terms   175
Helpful resources   193
Index   197

Preface

This handbook is written for anyone seeking to understand schizophrenia, whether a person with the illness, a family member, frontline health-care provider or student.

Schizophrenia tends to provoke anxiety for those who are unfamiliar with the current thinking about the illness or whose views about this illness are impacted by the considerable stereotyping, misconceptions and stigma associated with this illness. We have distilled key aspects of the current understanding and treatment of this illness and have organized them into 19 chapters. Each chapter is more or less self-contained (although there are some unavoidable repetitions), so that the reader can go directly to the relevant chapter. We neither pretend nor intend to answer all questions about this very complex illness. However, we have supplied several online and printed resources for those seeking additional information. In writing this book, we also kept in mind those who are curious about more recent research on schizophrenia, including mental-health students. We believe that this book will also be of value to educators and health policymakers whose business it is to dispel common myths about psychiatric disorders.

The practical advice and suggestions in this book are based on our own decades-long clinical and teaching experience, and largely consistent with current psychiatric practice. We use case examples, mnemonics and easy-to-use summary tables of key aspects of diagnosis and treatment of schizophrenia. We have deliberately opted for brevity, as a means of quickly delivering these key points, allowing the reader to pursue more in-depth exploration at leisure.

If the practice principles in this book appear to contradict any situation experienced by individual patients within specific clinical settings, the care provider should make appropriate referrals using his or her clinical judgment.

MSK would like to thank Angie Mines for editorial assistance. He is also grateful to his wife Asha Keshavan, MD, for her unwavering support and helpful suggestions. VHS is grateful to the patients and staff at the Program for Specialized Treatment Early in Psychosis at the Connecticut Mental Health Center (CMHC). The clinical work upon which his contributions are based was funded by the State of Connecticut, Department of Mental Health and Addiction Services, but this publication does not express the views of the Department of Mental Health and Addiction Services or the State of Connecticut. RR is ever grateful for the years of steadfast support by his family.

Matcheri S. Keshavan MD
Vinod H. Srihari MD
Ravinder Reddy MD

chapter 1

What is and is not schizophrenia?

The term 'schizophrenia' was coined almost a century ago by the Swiss psychiatrist Eugen Bleuler. Because of a long tradition of scientific terms being derived from Greek, Bleuler combined σχιζω (*schizo*, split or divide) and φρενος (*phrenos*, mind) to capture a split between the different 'psychic functions' of perception, thinking and feeling. Schizophrenia does not refer to a split personality.

Before considering what schizophrenia is, it is important to grasp the concept of psychosis, because it is central to the definition of schizophrenia.

Psychosis is best thought of as a *syndrome*, or a collection of symptoms (subjective experiences) and signs (observable behaviors) elicited by trained clinicians. Identifying psychosis is analogous to identifying fever. Just as fever results from an ongoing disturbance of temperature regulation, psychosis results from brain dysfunction. Fever has many causes, and so does psychosis.

Psychosis is a syndrome characterized by one or more of a variety of symptoms and signs that can be classified as reality distortion (delusions, hallucinations) or disorganization (in thought, behavior or expression of feeling).

All formal definitions of schizophrenia (two of which are widely used – the Diagnostic and Statistical Manual, 5th edition [DSM-5], and International Classification of Diseases, 11th revision [ICD-11]) require the presence of psychosis. However, it is important to remember that the presence of psychosis *alone* does not make for a diagnosis of schizophrenia. Individuals with schizophrenia additionally demonstrate a lack of motivation, reduction in spontaneous speech and social withdrawal (*negative symptoms*),

DOI: 10.4324/9781315152806-1

deficits in cognitive ability and disturbances in mood regulation that each or in combination can contribute to overall disability.

Psychosis is seen in a wide variety of disorders. In some, it is integral to the definition of the disorder. In other conditions, psychosis is neither essential to the diagnosis nor is it always present.

There is a long list of non-psychiatric conditions (see Chapter 5) in which psychosis can occur. Table 1.1 gives a list of *psychiatric* disorders in which psychosis occurs.

Table 1.1 Psychiatric disorders associated with psychosis

Disorders in which psychosis is integral to the definition	*Psychosis may be present but not essential to define the disorder*
Schizophrenia	Delirium
Schizophreniform Disorder	Dementia
Brief Psychotic Disorder	Mood disorders
Schizoaffective Disorder	Borderline Personality Disorder
Delusional Disorder	Substance-related disorders
Shared Psychotic Disorder	

The sufferers

Schizophrenia is a common illness, with a lifetime prevalence near 1% (Jauhar et al., 2022). Approximately 24 million individuals worldwide suffer from schizophrenia (WHO statistics). In the USA, there are approximately 2.6 million individuals diagnosed with schizophrenia. It is estimated that about one-third or more individuals with schizophrenia have not been in treatment for the past 12 months.

The direct costs of the illness, that is, the cost of caring for these patients, in the USA alone exceeds $62 billion per year. The total costs, including indirect costs such as productivity loss, may well exceed $280 billion per year (Schizophrenia & Psychosis Action Alliance, 2020).

Of approximately 600,000 homeless individuals in the USA, nearly three-fourths have a substance abuse disorder or mental illness, with a substantial proportion suffering from schizophrenia or related severe mental illness (Gutwinski et al., 2021).

The longevity of persons with schizophrenia is reduced by an average of 15 years, due to both unnatural (suicide, accidents) and, more commonly, natural causes (such as cardiovascular diseases). About 2% of patients with schizophrenia commit suicide over their lifetime, and this is at least ten times higher than the risk in the general population (Dutta et al., 2010).

The myths

Myths are a means of understanding the world and our place in it. Schizophrenia, like epilepsy before it, has been viewed as being 'un-understandable', and therefore evokes myths as explanations. Myths, like ignorance, can lead to troubling consequences – stigma and denial. The best way to counter ignorance is by education.

We suggest asking patients and their families about *their* understanding of schizophrenia, so that any misunderstanding of schizophrenia can be addressed directly. In all instances it is our *duty* to provide education about the best current understanding of schizophrenia and its treatment. Some of the common myths encountered and your potential responses are listed in Table 1.2.

The stigma of schizophrenia

Stigma is a negative attitude or idea about a person associated with social disapproval. Stigma can come from media (e.g. portrayals in film, television), cultural and family prejudice or institutional bias. Individuals with schizophrenia may also internalize these negative views (self-stigma). Schizophrenia is among the most stigmatized of all mental illnesses. A recent, large US study showed that over the last two decades, stigma for some psychiatric illnesses such as depression has been declining, but unfortunately this is not the case for schizophrenia. Rather, public perceptions attributing dangerousness to schizophrenia have actually increased (Pescosolido et al., 2021).

Today, we understand schizophrenia to mean an illness that impairs thinking, feeling and the ability to accurately perceive reality – it affects the whole individual. It can cause ANGUISH (Table 1.3) and cripple the individual, deeply affect his or her family and deprive the community of a fully participant member.

Table 1.2 A sampling of common and widespread myths about schizophrenia

Common and widespread myth	Your response
It is 'split personality'	A very common misunderstanding due to the origin of the word (*schizo*, split + *phrenia*, mind). It is not multiple personality disorder.
It only runs in families	It is true that there is a genetic contribution to schizophrenia, but a substantial number of patients have no family history of the illness.
Patients are violent or dangerous	There is some increase in incidence of violent behavior among individuals with schizophrenia, but this is very variable (Whiting et al., 2022). Individuals with schizophrenia are more likely to be victims of violence than the general population. However, some individuals with schizophrenia act aggressively as a result of the psychosis, particularly paranoia.
There is no effective treatment	There are very effective treatments, although responses to treatment vary greatly.
It is due to bad parenting, especially by the mother	Several decades ago, the so-called *schizophrenogenic mother* was held responsible. There is no evidence that bad parenting causes schizophrenia, although parents can play a significant role in illness management.
It is due to drug abuse	Drug abuse is very common in individuals with schizophrenia, particularly at the onset of illness. There is evidence that drug abuse can precipitate psychosis, though it is unclear whether it causes schizophrenia. Substance abuse can interfere with treatment.
It is their fault	It is not the fault of the patient. No one chooses to have schizophrenia!
Children don't get it	Although schizophrenia typically emerges in late adolescence and adulthood, it can appear in early life (childhood schizophrenia). Treatment is similar to adult schizophrenia.
Marriage 'cures' schizophrenia	In some cultures it is believed that marriage cures schizophrenia. There is no evidence for this. While the possibility exists that marriage may have beneficial effects (due to a caring partner), a dysfunctional marriage can be problematic.

Evil spirits cause schizophrenia	In some communities there are strong beliefs about supernatural causes of suffering. It is best to work with, rather than against, these beliefs. Our approach is to suggest that conventional (modern) treatments can work alongside efforts to cast off evil spirits, so that patients are not forced to choose the non-medical approach.
Patients are 'possessed'	This is analogous to 'evil spirits' but not identical. Possession can occur with 'spirits' of all sorts – good, bad or neutral. The same approach as above is recommended.
Past misdeeds cause it	In cultures where belief in past lives exists, present suffering is attributed to past actions, usually 'sins'. Our approach is to suggest to patients and their families that the best we can do is rectify the suffering in the present.
Only rituals cure schizophrenia	This is one of the most challenging myths to deal with because individuals and families who utilize traditional rituals will try these first before seeking medical help. This results in longer duration of untreated psychosis, which is a risk factor for poor outcome.
A spell has been cast	Similar to other supernatural attributions for schizophrenia, being under a spell is quite common. In addition to problems of engaging patients into treatment, there is a risk that patients or their families may retaliate against the spell-caster, if known.
They are stupid	The thinking disturbance of schizophrenia can be mistaken for 'stupidity'. It is important to avoid negative terms such as stupidity.
A person with schizophrenia is blessed and holy	The only benefit of this myth is that the patient tends not to be mistreated. However, there can be reluctance in seeking treatment.
Treatment is lifelong	Once diagnosis of schizophrenia is made with certainty, treatment may continue for a lifetime. However, if patients remain symptom-free for long periods of time, lowering the dose of medications may be tried.
Schizophrenia is a social construction and a harmful label	All medical diagnoses are constructions to help identify illness and direct care in a manner that is specific to the illness and centered on the patient's needs. While unacceptable stigma can become attached to a diagnostic label, this should not mean that no identifiable illness exists. A lack of diagnostic identification usually has led to other, less useful constructions (e.g. possession by evil spirits, poor parenting) that not only are inaccurate accounts of causes but cause unnecessary suffering.

Table 1.3 Consequences of stigma (ANGUISH)

Aloneness	Patients, as well as their families, suffer in silence. This can lead to social isolation. There is also a tendency to 'cover up' the illness.
Negative experiences	Patients will suffer all sorts of negative experiences. Name-calling, inability to complete school work, no job offers, losing friends, being asked to leave business establishments, and so on.
Guilt and shame	These feelings are commonly experienced by patients and families, leading to distorted perceptions of self.
Untreated illness duration	Increased duration of untreated illness is a strong predictor of poor outcome.
Incarceration	Because of untreated illness, disturbing behaviors can result in legal trouble, and such individuals can be lost to psychiatric care for long periods of time. Increasingly, enlightened legal systems are recognizing mental illness in their inmates and providing treatment.
Substance abuse	Illicit drugs and alcohol are often used to deal with the psychological pain, leading to their own set of problems.
Health worsens	Avoidance or lack of healthcare access also contributes to poorer physical health.

Summary

- The term 'schizophrenia' was coined to capture the notion of a 'fractured' or 'shattered' mind, not *split mind*.
- Psychosis is a state characterized by loss of contact with reality.
- Not all psychosis is schizophrenia, but schizophrenia is a form of psychosis.
- Approximately 50 million individuals worldwide suffer from schizophrenia. The suffering and economic costs are enormous.
- Many homeless individuals are mentally ill, and about half suffer from schizophrenia.
- Stigma has powerful negative effects and should be combated.
- Myths about schizophrenia are numerous and found worldwide. They are associated with stigma and denial of illness. Stigma should be combated vigorously by education.

References

Dutta, R., Murray, R. M., Hotopf, M., Allardyce, J., Jones, P. B., & Boydell, J. (2010). Reassessing the long-term risk of suicide after a first episode of psychosis. *Archives of General Psychiatry, 67*, 1230–1237.

Gutwinski, S., Schreiter, S., Deutscher, K., & Fazel, S. (2021, August 23). The prevalence of mental disorders among homeless people in high-income countries: An updated systematic review and meta-regression analysis. *PLoS Medicine, 18*(8).

Jauhar, S., Johnstone, M., & McKenna, P. J. (2022, January 29). Schizophrenia. *Lancet, 399*(10323), 473–486.

Pescosolido, B. A., Halpern-Manners, A., Luo, L., & Perry, B. (2021, December 1). Trends in public stigma of mental illness in the US, 1996–2018. *JAMA Network Open, 4*(12).

Schizophrenia & Psychosis Action Alliance. (2020). Schizophrenia (WHO. int) Schizophrenia cost the U.S. $281.6 billion in 2020 – Schizophrenia & Psychosis Action Alliance (sczaction.org).

Whiting, D., Gulati, G., Geddes, J. R., & Fazel, S. (2022, February 1). Association of schizophrenia spectrum disorders and violence perpetration in adults and adolescents from 15 countries: A systematic review and meta-analysis. *JAMA Psychiatry, 79*(2), 120–132.

chapter 2

Assessment of schizophrenia

Assessing the clinical state of patients with a psychotic disorder can be challenging, unintuitive and frustrating. This is due to the nature of the illness. Communication with patients experiencing psychosis can be hampered by the presence of thinking difficulties, delusions and hallucinations. This is true, in fact, for all disorders that are accompanied by psychotic phenomena.

Interviewing a patient with psychosis can be an anxiety-provoking experience for the novice. Patients are frequently uncooperative or outright hostile. Alternatively, they may be cooperative but unable to communicate effectively.

Most importantly, remember that the person in front of you is *not* a 'psychotic' or a 'schizophrenic', however convenient these labels might be; rather, you are interacting with an individual suffering *from* a psychotic disorder, just as you or I might suffer from cancer or an intellectual disability. (We wouldn't like to be referred to as cancerous or retarded!) Remembering this will ease the fear and frustrations one may experience while interviewing patients with psychosis.

Observe experienced clinicians interviewing patients with psychotic disorders. If possible, interview patients *without* psychosis a few times prior to interviewing patients with psychosis. You will feel more practiced in your interview method.

While interviewing *any* patient, it is important to:

- be non-judgmental
- be patient

DOI: 10.4324/9781315152806-2

- use vocabulary familiar to the patient (no jargon)
- inquire about the details of the history
- offer hope and support

EMPATHY is a quality whereby it is perceived by the patient that the interviewer has a genuine appreciation of his or her distress. Empathy (putting oneself 'in the shoes of the other person') cannot be 'manufactured' or pretended for any length of time. The best expression of empathy is genuine caring about the patient and his or her problems through sensitive and detailed understanding of the issues. No amount of 'empathetic noises' such as, 'That must have been terrible', or 'I understand', can substitute for genuine empathy. While *sympathy* (feeling sorry for others) has a role in interviewing, overdoing it is counterproductive.

HUMOR can be a useful tool in assessing mental state or facilitating therapeutic alliance, but there is significant risk of a misfired moment during an interview – or worse, a joke or humorous turn of phrase being misconstrued. Smiling at something humorous said or done by the patient is fine if it was intended to be funny, but beware of uncontrolled guffaws!

Interviewing an individual suspected of experiencing psychosis

Allow the patient to tell his or her story. If the patient is silent or unwilling to talk, begin by asking about their understanding of why they are at this place now or about the trip to the clinic or hospital, or about their living situation.

A lot can be learned by listening to the initial verbalization. The flow of speech can reveal thinking disturbances (is the thinking linear or disordered?). The construction of the speech can betray aphasias or disturbances in logic. Delusions can become apparent by the content of the speech (statements about being spied upon by police cameras, for example).

Think of the interview as a series of **OLA** ('hello' in Spanish):

Observe behavior.
Listen especially to spontaneous verbalization.
Ask open-ended, leading or follow-up questions as required.

Even if the focus of the interview is psychosis, make sure to ask about other conditions to ensure a comprehensive diagnostic assessment.

How much to ask and when?

All interviews are conducted within a set of constraints:

- time (the amount of time practicably available)
- location (emergency room, inpatient unit, outpatient service)
- patient's capacity to communicate (verbal, guarded, rambling or mute)
- risky behaviors (aggressive, violent, acutely suicidal)

Your task is to discover the most salient information relevant to the goal of the interview. If you anticipate hospitalization, consider what kinds of information you'd like to have immediately and what information can be gathered later. For example, for an acutely suicidal patient, gathering family history may not be the most important task at this time. If the patient is seeking transfer of outpatient care, likely you'll want specific information to assure smooth transition of care, such as reason for transfer, recent course of treatment and so forth.

That said, at a minimum you need to determine whether the patient is dangerous to self or others (reviewed in Chapter 14), is using illicit substances, is adherent with treatment if previously treated and whether there is any ongoing medical problem.

> JB is being seen at a busy emergency service because of incessant suicidal thoughts. You have no previous medical notes because she has not been seen at this hospital before.

The questions you definitely want to ask:

Have you attempted suicide before? Past suicide attempts are a strong predictor of suicide.

Is anyone in your family depressed? This gives you an indication that depression may be familial. It will not necessarily help with estimating current risk of suicide; instead ask about suicide in relatives, a better predictor of suicide.

Are the voices commanding you to do something? Auditory hallucinations commanding harm to self can be incessant and patients can 'give in' to the voices.

Are you taking any medicine? This can tell you about whether the patient is in treatment, level of medication adherence and whether there is access to medications with overdose potential.

Do you live alone? Living alone is a risk factor for suicide.

> AK, a 17-year-old, comes to the clinic accompanied by his mother. She made this first appointment because of her concerns that AK is isolating himself, he sometimes laughs for no apparent reason, his mood is erratic and he stays up all night.

The following questions will go a long way in helping arrive at a working diagnosis:

Is AK using drugs? Practically all substances of abuse are associated with altered behavior, including psychosis.

Is AK experiencing hallucinations? Hallucinations are a common psychotic phenomenon, particularly in schizophrenia.

How is AK doing in school? This can be a valuable indicator of how AK's functioning has been affected by recent changes in behavior. Decline in functioning is one of the criteria for diagnostic threshold for many psychiatric disorders, including schizophrenia.

Does anyone in the family have schizophrenia? If there is a family history of schizophrenia, it allows estimation of risk of a psychotic disorder but does not provide diagnostic certainty.

Manner of questioning

There are many techniques and strategies that are available in the service of eliciting information. With practice one can learn how and when to apply them appropriately. Conducting lots of interviews and watching experienced interviewers can greatly enhance one's skills. The basic types of question are:

- open-ended (*how have you been feeling?*)
- leading (*you've been feeling poorly lately, haven't you?*)
- closed-ended (*are you depressed?*)

It is usually a good idea to start with open-ended questions to obtain unbiased information, and then to follow up with closed-ended questions as needed. Patients with psychotic disorders often require closed-ended and leading questions to move the interview along and to gather information. This is usually due to cognitive deficits and negative symptoms. Paranoia also can significantly impair the flow of information.

A rule of thumb is not to challenge the belief by which the patient holds the delusions. It is worth reasoning with the patient about weakly held delusions if the patient is willing to discuss them, but strongly held delusions are best addressed by passively acknowledging and neither challenging nor agreeing with them. A common fear is that agreeing to a delusion will further entrench the delusional thinking. Recall the definition of a delusion – a belief that is held in spite of evidence to the contrary. Remember, though, that you do not have to condone the content of the delusions.

Imagining psychosis

Unlike depression or anxiety, our ability to genuinely understand psychotic phenomena is limited. However, it is important to try to *imagine* what a psychotic experience may be like for the patient. Put yourself in their 'shoes': imagine what it might feel like to be spied upon constantly or to have persecutory voices tormenting you. Such an exercise will not only help you to phrase questions in helpful ways and assist patients to articulate their experiences, but also engender empathy. It is quite common for patients with schizophrenia to have difficulty in describing psychotic phenomena or not be fully forthcoming about the effect of psychosis on their lives. One of our favorite phrases during interviewing is, 'I wonder . . .'.

> *I wonder whether you keep a weapon nearby in case the people trying to hurt you or break into your apartment.*
>
> *I wonder whether the voices that bother you say really awful things about you, things that you would never reveal to anyone.*
>
> *I wonder whether you feel like you don't fit in because of your illness.*
>
> *If I thought that others could read my mind, I might be forced to stop having thoughts that they could pick up. I wonder if you feel that way.*

We have found this approach to be very useful in getting patients to talk about the distress they experience. We do refrain from using this approach in patients who are experiencing severe thought broadcasting (i.e. the sense that others can read one's thoughts) because they experience these questions as validation of their psychotic experience, which can lead to further distress.

Mental status examination

The mental status examination (MSE), analogous to a physical examination, is a process by which the clinician investigates mental functioning. The history and MSE constitute a psychiatric examination. In theory, the MSE is performed after obtaining a comprehensive history. In reality the MSE occurs in conjunction with obtaining the history, beginning the moment the patient is seen, even before any conversation occurs. A proper mental status exam will have the following components we call the 'A-to-J' of MSE:

- Appearance
- Behavior
- Conversation – to listen to the *form* of thinking
- Delusions – to listen to the *content* of thinking
- Emotions – mood and affect
- Faculties – higher faculties such as attention and orientation
- General intelligence
- Hallucinations
- Insight
- Judgment

Assessing the major components of psychosis

Psychosis is most commonly established by the presence of delusions, hallucinations or thought disorder. Additionally, patients present with emotional, behavioral, cognitive and neurological disturbances that accompany psychosis.

Mr. O reports he is concerned that his wife has been having an affair for the past several months. He thinks this because she doesn't answer her phone at work and returns home smelling 'funny'. He follows her and has hired an investigator to confirm this. Despite no evidence, he remains convinced that she is unfaithful.

Is the patient delusional? If so, how do you define a delusion? Mr. O is clearly suspicious of his wife's fidelity. To determine a delusion, more questions need to be asked to determine if his concerns are plausible or are based on 'flimsy' evidence. If the evidence presented appears implausible, then a delusion should be suspected. However, it is necessary to challenge Mr. O's assumptions in order to determine how firmly these beliefs are held. For example, one could ask, 'is it possible, for sake of argument, that you are mistaken about your wife actually having an affair?' Not allowing for even the possibility that he may be mistaken strengthens the case for the presence of a delusion (of jealousy).

Delusions

Delusions are fixed, false beliefs that are held in spite of evidence to the contrary, are at odds with the community's cultural and religious beliefs, are inconsistent with the level of education of the patient and can be patently irrational. Overvalued ideas are beliefs which are less firmly held than delusions and tend to be less irrational; they are more easily challenged.

Delusions can be well-organized with ideas connected to each other (systematized delusions), or non-systematized and fragmented. It is not uncommon for patients also to have intense preoccupation with esoteric and vague ideas about philosophical, religious, or psychological themes. Hypochondriacal thinking about unlikely and bizarre medical conditions may also occur. Delusions can be about any sort of idea, but the most common ones are listed in Table 2.1.

Table 2.1 Common delusions

Term	Observations in patients
Paranoid	Feeling persecuted; feeling taken advantage of; conspiracy of harm or spying; messages in innocuous events

Table 2.1 Continued

Grandiose	Unique or superior abilities; special powers; superior personage
Somatic	Sense that something is uniquely wrong with the body that has not been or cannot be detected by others
Erotomanic	Convinced that someone famous, beautiful, rich or otherwise beyond reach is in love with the patient; also known as de Clérambault's syndrome
Jealous	Sometimes referred to as the Othello syndrome; the patient is convinced that a spouse or partner is cheating
Thought insertion	Belief or experience that outside forces or entities place thoughts into one's mind
Thought broadcasting	Belief or experience that one's thoughts are broadcast to the external world and may be 'read' by others
Referential thinking	Also called ideas of reference, wherein the individual interprets common events as having personal relevance (e.g. messages from the TV or songs, or innocuous gestures signifying specific codes)
Delusions of passivity	A sense that the mind or body is being controlled or interfered with by external forces or persons

How do we discover that a patient is delusional?

It is not helpful to ask, *'are you delusional?'* One way to begin is to ask, *'do you have unusual ideas that others don't agree with?'* Delusional thinking can be picked up by listening to what the patient is expressing, particularly their concerns. Not infrequently, though, patients will not divulge their thoughts spontaneously. In such cases, it is useful to ask rather directly: in other words, **OLA** (observe, listen, ask).

By listening carefully, one can get clues about delusional thinking. The trick is to follow up with questions that can sensitively probe further.

Patient: I had to take two buses to get here. You'd think that they'd at least let me sit down. By the way, can I have bus tokens to get back home? I used my last tokens on that stupid bus.

Is there anything worthwhile following up in this statement? It would be useful to inquire about the events on the bus. The patient is clearly upset about something he experienced on the 'stupid' bus.

Hallucinations

Hallucinations are false perceptions (Table 2.2). These occur in the *absence* of a stimulus, and can involve any of the bodily sensations (seeing, hearing, smelling, tasting and feeling).

Illusions, on the other hand, are *misinterpretations* of actual stimuli. Illusions are not typically considered psychotic phenomena, although they are commonly experienced by patients with schizophrenia.

The most common hallucination in schizophrenia is auditory (70–80% of patients). The presence of visual or olfactory hallucinations alone should raise suspicion of underlying medical or neurological disorder.

How do we discover that a patient is experiencing hallucinations?
Unlike in the case of delusions, it is usually a good idea to ask directly about hallucinations if not already divulged by the patient. For example, one could ask:

Have you ever heard sounds or voices in your head or even from the outside that you couldn't quite figure out? Have you ever heard voices that other people didn't hear?

Have you seen things or had visions that didn't quite fit with what was going on at the time? Did you ever see things or people that others couldn't see at the same time?

What about feelings or sensations in your body that were different from your usual experiences?

Have you smelled or tasted anything unusual – it could be nice, like perfume, or bad, like burning flesh, or some taste like metal?

Table 2.2 Hallucinations

Term	Observations in patients
Auditory	Hearing sounds; unintelligible whispers; single words (such as a name) or sentences; single or multiple familiar or unfamiliar voices; comments on patient's actions; conversing among speakers; voices commanding actions, including harm to others and self, or sexual acts (command hallucinations); varying loudness; commonly worse when alone; patients talking to self usually in response to auditory hallucinations

Table 2.2 Continued

Visual	Seeing shadows at the corner of eye; ghost-like images; natural and unnatural objects; partial or complete images of known or unknown persons; complete scenes of events, commonly disturbing images
Somatosensory	Transient sensations of pain, electricity or movement; sensations that body parts are moving, including the brain; shrinking of body parts; alterations in shape, color or texture of body parts, including skin
Olfactory	Usually unpleasant smells (such as feces, burning rubber or flesh), but occasionally pleasant smells like perfume or fruits
Gustatory	Unusual tastes, particularly metallic or salty

Thought disturbance

The structure of thinking is reflected in speech and writing and in behavior. Disordered thinking is common in schizophrenia and takes on many forms. The end result of thought disorder is impaired communication (see below).

Clinician: *How are you feeling today?*

Patient: *Fine, doc. But these humanoids really suck. The universe is particulate. I just wish they'd stop squeezing my intestines. How are you, doc?* (Smiling)

Here patient is exhibiting loss of association, neologism ('the universe is particulate') and inappropriate affect.

Thought disturbance can be so subtle that it doesn't interfere with most communication, or so severe that speech is unintelligible. Common types of thought disorder are listed in Table 2.3 and Figure 2.1.

Table 2.3 Thought-process disturbance

Term	*Observations in patients*
Circumstantiality	Speech is over-inclusive with detail; thoughts start off linearly, but then wander off for a while, returning later to the original point. In order to detect circumstantiality, it is important to allow the patient to speak for a period of time before interrupting

Tangentiality	Thoughts start off linearly, but quickly veer off into unrelated areas without returning to the original point. When interrupted, patients tend to ask what the question was in the first place
Loose associations	There is an apparent disconnection between one thought (usually a sentence) and the next. An indication that loosening of associations is occurring is when the interviewer is unable to follow the train of thought ('huh?'). When severe, speech becomes incomprehensible
Thought blocking	In mid-sentence the patient appears to have lost the train of thought. However, you need to ascertain whether the patient actually 'lost' the thought – true thought blocking – or was distracted by competing thoughts
Flight of ideas	This represents a combination of thought disorders. Here a fairly complete idea is followed by another idea with only a tenuous or no connection between these thoughts. One experiences it as a zigzagging through conversation
Neologism	Coining of new terms with idiosyncratic meanings (e.g. 'flushistic')
Perseveration	Persistent repetition of a response to new and unrelated stimuli
Verbigeration	Persistent repetition of words or phrases (e.g. 'I was going the corrected way. They hadn't corrected the signs, and now I was lost and had to get corrected directions'.)
Word salad	Complete lack of meaningful connections between words (e.g. 'seeing blasts tin hatched flour all along'). This thought disturbance is quite rare

How do we discover that a patient has a thought disorder?

Unlike assessment of hallucinations or delusions, thought disorder is best detected by listening. Open-ended questions are the most effective for eliciting thought disorder.

To determine *past* thought disorder, in the absence of medical records or corroborative information, it is useful to ask the patient something like:

Was there a time in the past when people complained that they couldn't quite follow what you were saying?

Have you ever noticed that your thinking was muddled?

Did you ever notice that, in the middle of a thought, it just sort of disappeared and you couldn't recall it?

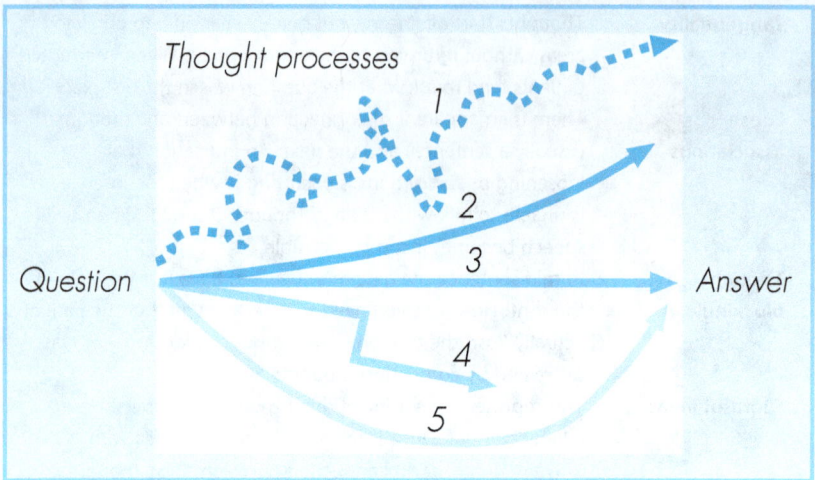

1) Loss of associations
2) Tangentiality
3) Linear thinking
4) Flight of ideas
5) Circumstantiality

Figure 2.1 A schematic diagram to reflect linear thinking and types of thought disorder.

Negative symptoms

In addition to psychosis, patients with schizophrenia commonly exhibit negative symptoms. These are a constellation of signs and symptoms that are characterized by diminution or loss of functioning (Table 2.4). This is in contrast to **positive symptoms** (hallucinations and delusions) which reflect augmentation or addition of functioning.

Negative symptoms are classified as *primary* (due to the illness itself) or *secondary* (consequence of the illness or its treatment). The importance of this distinction lies in their treatment (see Chapter 9). Negative symptoms can be especially bothersome to patients and are often resistant to treatment (Figure 2.1).

Disturbances of emotion

Patients with schizophrenia present with a variety of emotional states – anxiety, perplexity, elation or depression. Expansive mood may present as ecstasy or exaltation (sometimes confused with religious experiences). Inappropriate affect, which is the disconnection between the display of emotion and the

Table 2.4 Negative symptoms (the 'five As')

Term	Function affected	Observations in patients
Alogia	Fluency of speech	Reduced quantity of speech; brief answers to questions; monosyllabic responses, such as 'yes' or 'no'
Affective blunting	Emotional expression	Reduced range of facial and body movement, classified as restricted, blunted and flat (mild, moderate and severe, respectively); sitting in a chair with little movement
Avolition	Volition and drive	Frequently confused with laziness because patients have difficulty initiating or following through on tasks; inability to plan for the future
Anhedonia	Hedonic capacity	Inability to enjoy activities previously found pleasurable, including intimacy; performing tasks in a mechanical, bored manner; staring at the television for hours with no indication of enjoyment
Asociality	Social interactions	Tendency to isolate

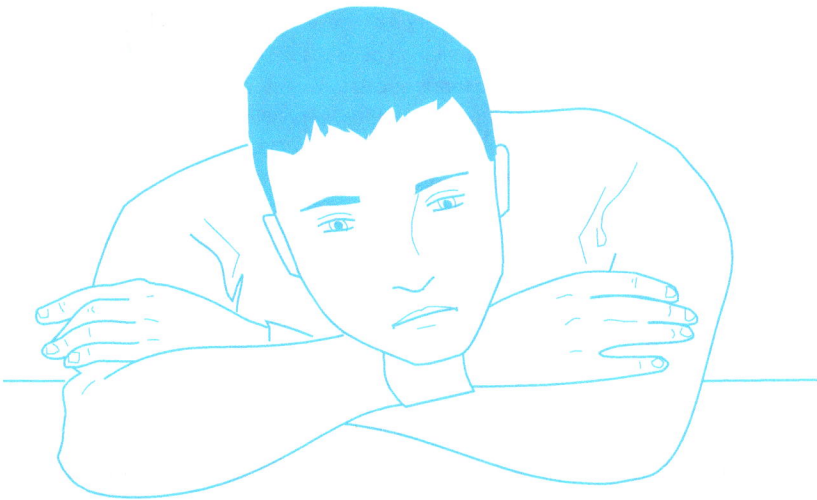

Figure 2.2 The depressive appearance.

thought and speech content, is quite common (e.g. the patient may grin while describing a sad event, or burst into tears while describing an amusing situation).

Behavioral disturbances

Schizophrenia patients frequently manifest psychomotor and behavioral abnormalities (Table 2.5). These behaviors are not necessarily a consequence of underlying delusions or hallucinations.

Cognitive abnormalities

There has been increasing focus on cognition (higher intellectual functioning including awareness, perception, reasoning, memory and problem-solving) in schizophrenia. Advances in cognitive neurosciences have significantly bolstered our understanding of the nature of cognitive disturbances in schizophrenia, and treatments are being developed to remediate these deficits (Table 2.6).

Table 2.5 Behavioral disturbances

Term	Observations in patients
Posturing	The assumption of odd postures
Mannerisms	Goal-directed behaviors carried out in an odd or stilted fashion
Stereotypies	Non-purposeful and uniformly repetitive motions, such as tapping and rocking
Echopraxia	The repetitive imitation of movements performed by others
Echolalia	The repetitive imitation of words or statements made by others
Catatonia	There are two forms of catatonia – stuporous and excited. Catatonic stupor presents as immobility, posturing (waxy flexibility), mutism and negativity. Echolalia and echopraxia may also be seen. Catatonic excitement presents as excited and aimless motor activity

Table 2.6 Cognitive deficits

Domain	Function affected	Observations in patients
Attention	Ability to focus on specific aspects of the environment while excluding others	Distractibility, inability to stay on task

Perception and recognition		Missing the point of conversation
Memory	Working memory, verbal learning and memory, visual learning and memory	Impaired recall of facts, stories, ideas
Language	Perception, processing and production of language	Impaired syntax, vocabulary and speech output
Executive functions	Problem-solving, planning, reasoning	Deficits in planning, sequencing of actions, concept formation, mental-set shifting and selective attention

Neurological abnormalities

Patients with schizophrenia can have subtle neurologic disturbances, referred to as 'soft signs', which consist of disturbances in **motor coordination** (gait, balance, coordination and muscle tone), **sensory integration** (graphesthesia, stereognosis and proprioception) and **primitive reflexes** (such as the palmomental, grasp and snout reflexes). While these findings clearly substantiate the biological basis of schizophrenia, they do not necessarily help us with the diagnosis of this illness.

Summary (see also Table 2.7)

- The interview is a process of observation, listening and asking questions.
- All interviews are conducted within a set of constraints, but at a minimum determine whether the patient is dangerous to self or others, is using illicit substances and is compliant with treatment, and whether there are any ongoing medical problems.
- Interviewing a patient with psychosis can be an anxiety-provoking experience for the novice. Remembering the person in front of you is *not* a 'psychotic', but an individual suffering *from* a psychotic disorder, will ease the fear and frustration.
- While interviewing it is important to remain nonjudgmental, patient and plain-speaking (no jargon) and to offer hope and support.
- When interviewing an individual suspected of experiencing psychosis, allow the patient to tell his or her story.
- A lot can be learned by listening to the initial speech; thinking disturbances can be revealed and delusions may become apparent by the content of the speech.

Table 2.7 Assessment strategies

The issue	What to do
Uncovering delusions	First listen – the manner and content of the verbalizations will offer many clues to delusional thinking; then probe sensitively about the details of the delusions and their effect on the patient's life; do not challenge the delusion
Uncovering hallucinations	Observe first – does the patient appear distracted, as if attending to some inner voices or visions; is the patient mumbling or talking to self aloud? If required, ask directly about hallucinatory experiences
Uncovering thought disorder	Listen; don't interrupt prematurely; ensure that the patient understood the question correctly so as not to mislabel the response!
Negative symptoms	Observe facial expression, particularly in response to material that could elicit feelings; note whether gestures are used and the body's posture; ask about pleasurable activities; ask about future plans; ask about the week's activities
The angry patient	There are many reasons why patients present with anger – there may be situational reasons, such as being brought in against their will, or it may be due to underlying paranoia or irritability. The first order of business is to ensure everyone's safety. A patient who is helped to feel safe is less likely to remain angry or act out aggressively. Acknowledge the patient's anger. Enquire whether the patient would like food or water. If the patient begins to shout, it is alright to state that the shouting is interfering with your ability to help the patient.
The paranoid patient	The issue is one of trusting the interviewer. Sometimes it helps to ally with the emotional response to (rather than the truth claims of) a delusion to gain trust. It is possible to join the patient in their fear of turning on their TV because they want to avoid the distress of attending to messages from figures on the screen, and express empathy with their frustration at missing their favorite shows. One might even join them in their frustration at the forces lined up against them. The 'us against them' approach is useful, but you can do this without agreeing with the content of the delusional belief. Additionally, the patient may incorporate you into the delusional system, so you must understand what role you play in it and adjust your approach accordingly.

chapter 3

Social determinants of health affecting assessment

A variety of factors can affect the clinical presentation and treatment of psychotic disorders. These factors, many of which are social determinants of health (SDoH), can modify the clinical picture as well as the outcome of treatment. Thus, assessment and treatment planning must take these factors into account. For details regarding SdoH that impact schizophrenia, the reader is referred to the review by Jester et al. (2023).

One view is that all peoples of the world are essentially biologically similar, particularly with regard to brain functioning. Thus, with the exception of a few minor differences, schizophrenia and related psychotic disorders essentially ought to be the similar across the world. This view was supported by landmark studies by the World Health Organization (WHO) in the 1970s. The International Pilot Study of Schizophrenia (Sartorius et al., 1974) found that the clinical presentation of schizophrenia was similar across the ten countries studied (Figure 3.1).

On the other hand, there has been increasing appreciation that sociocultural factors can shape individual worldviews and perceptions and affect illness presentation, attribution of meaning to the illness experience and the outcomes of treatment. The same WHO studies that noted similarities in the clinical presentation of schizophrenia across continents found significant differences in treatment outcome. Contrary to expectations, patients from developing countries like India and Nigeria fared better than patients from the USA and UK. Some have argued that the better outcomes measured in developing countries stem from the nature of the subjects who enrolled in the study and remained available for outcomes monitoring. Nevertheless, these and other studies have raised awareness of the potential impact

DOI: 10.4324/9781315152806-3

of broader social, cultural and environmental determinants of treatment response and broader health outcomes. These should be considered during clinical assessment and treatment.

RC is a 31-year-old woman of South Asian origin who lives alone; she recently moved overseas for postgraduate studies. She is referred to the clinic because of her insistent complaints that the male professors are giving her failing grades because she is smarter than them. She is certain because she hears them talking about her brilliance and her 'foreign' looks.

Which of the following factors may be important in RC's presentation? Why?
a) Educational achievements
b) Ethnicity
c) Immigration
d) Culture
e) Age

RC is a highly educated individual, but this in itself doesn't seem to have direct bearing on the clinical presentation. Ethnicity is an important consideration; recent research suggests that low ethnic density may be a significant risk factor. To clarify, risk of psychosis in minority group individuals is higher if the neighborhood-level proportion of others belonging to the same group is low. Immigration is frequently cited as a risk factor for schizophrenia. In the case of RC, inquiry about her mental state prior to arriving in the UK may be more important than assuming that voluntary immigration for educational purposes would necessarily increase stress and thereby precipitate psychosis. In all instances one must be sensitive to cultural factors when assessing patients from non-majority cultural backgrounds. With RC we would want to discover whether there are any culturally derived issues with regard to male professors. RC was 31 years old, an age consistent with the later age at onset of schizophrenia in females, relative to males.

An individual's '**LEGACIE**' can significantly influence the risk of developing schizophrenia spectrum disorders, the expression of the illness, the treatment response and the long-term clinical outcome. There is a long list of biological and non-biological factors that have a role in schizophrenia. Discussed below are factors that have been identified as important SdoH, some of which have been quite well-researched.

Location
Ethnicity

Gender
Age
Culture
Immigration
Environment

Gender

Sex and gender are not identical. Sex is designated at birth (*what you are born as:* biological male, female or intersex) while gender incorporates sex but involves the assumption of a broader social identity over the course of psychosocial development (*what you are born as and become*). There are several important distinctions between men and women with schizophrenia regarding the clinical picture, treatment response and long-term outcome. It has been theorized that these differences may be due to biological (e.g. estrogen) and environmental (e.g. better socialization in women) factors (Table 3.1).

Table 3.1 Gender differences

	Women	*Men*
Age at onset of illness	Onset five years later than men. Late-onset schizophrenia is more common in women	Earlier onset, in late teens and early adulthood
Onset of illness Clinical presentation	Rapid onset More commonly present with depressed mood, paranoia, fewer negative symptoms and better functioning while ill	Insidious onset More negative symptoms
Treatment response	More rapid and complete response to initial treatment. However, women are more likely to have side effects	A more gradual response, with persistence of symptoms, particularly negative symptoms
Long-term outcome	Better than men	Poorer than women, regardless of how outcome is defined
Sex-specific differences	Hormonal fluctuations can affect symptom severity	

Ethnicity and race

It was believed in the USA that there were greater rates of schizophrenia in black persons than white persons. A large study (Robins & Regier, 1991) in the USA did not find significant differences between the two groups. It has been thought that schizophrenia has roughly the same prevalence across the world, though this is increasingly debated. For example, the rates of schizophrenia in Afro-Caribbean immigrants in the UK appear to be significantly higher, perhaps due to the stress of emigration. There also are geographical 'pockets' of higher prevalence rates, as in northern Sweden and Finland, and western Ireland. See additional discussion in Chapter 17.

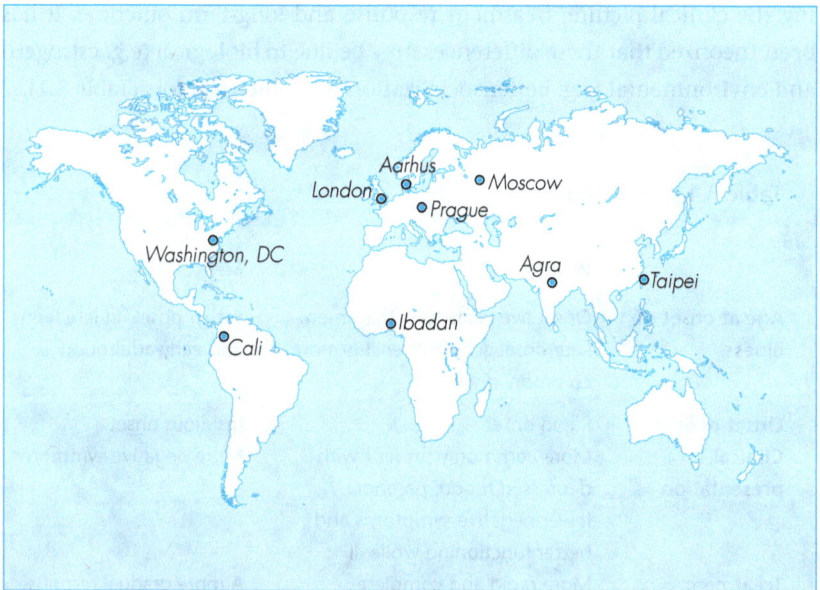

Figure 3.1 Centers where the International Pilot Study of Schizophrenia (Sartorius et al., 1974) was conducted.

Culture

Culture (Latin *colere*, to inhabit, to cultivate) is a term that has many meanings and has been used to explain or sometimes obscure the differences between individuals. A definition influential in early 20th-century anthropology – 'knowledge, belief, arts, morals, law, customs, and any other capabilities and habits acquired by man as a member of society' – illustrates how difficult it is to pin down this fluid concept. While a full discussion of the topic of culture and mental illness is beyond the scope of this chapter, listed in the Box are several ways in which this concept is invoked in assessments:

CULTURE
- Meanings, values and behavioral norms that are learned and transmitted in the dominant society and within its social groups
- Powerfully influences thinking, feelings and self-concept
- Defines normality and deviance
- Facilitates healthy adaptations
- Has mechanisms that facilitate conflict resolution
- Induces psychopathology by presenting stressors
- Reduces psychopathology by in-built protective factors
- Affects onset, course and outcome of illness, as well as acceptance of treatments
- Shapes tolerance for certain behaviors and clinical symptoms
- Shapes culture-specific expressions of distress

It is important to avoid the assumption of culture as a static, uninterrupted set of values or practices that somehow define the essence of a person (the fallacy of essentialism), when in fact cultures are dynamic, include much variation within any cultural category and are themselves routinely changed by individuals within and via interactions with others outside the cultural group. Also, as with other classifications (e.g. by race, gender, class), categorizing patients by their culture, while sometimes useful, carries the risk of prejudging their possibilities.

THE CLINICIAN'S CULTURAL COMPETENCY To offer our patients a sense of being understood, we must at a minimum be constantly vigilant of how our own cultural perceptions and expectations can color our clinical interactions. In addition, we need to be culturally aware. This doesn't mean becoming an expert on every culture you are likely to encounter in your practice. Rather, it means that you are inquisitive about other cultures, able to elicit viewpoints derived from unfamiliar cultural traditions and able to engage with these when they can enrich or hinder treatment. Given the complexities and the dynamically changing nature of these factors, cultural competency is more of a continuous journey than a destination. On the other hand, cultural humility as an attitude will increase your ability to elicit relevant cultural information, thereby improving care of your patients.

Immigration

Immigrants appear to be at heightened risk for developing schizophrenia. One view is that the increased risk is a consequence of stress associated with migration. The alternative view holds that the presence of mental illness itself promotes migration. The interaction between the migrant and the host country is a continuous process, rather than something that happens simply when borders are crossed. The nature of these stresses can also vary based on the circumstances driving the migration and the immigration-status categories, e.g. guest worker, refugee or student. Potential sources of stress include interactions with the new socioeconomic system, interactions with the host country's culture and changes in the social network of the migrant.

Questions to assess a migrant's experience are:

When did you come here? How old were you?
What were the reasons for moving?
Did you experience difficulties in getting here?
How big was the difference between your birth place and here?
Did you come here alone or in a group?
What are/were you feeling about the new culture?
Did people here help you adjust?
Did/do you feel accepted here?
What was your life like before you came here?

Asking such questions can go a long way towards acknowledging migrants' challenges in adapting to their new (temporary or permanent) home, validating the complex set of emotions they experience as a result of migration. Sadly, there is an assumption that if individuals *choose* to migrate, they ought not to complain about problems. Unfortunately, some immigrants hold the same view and consequently suffer needlessly. An additional burden that immigrants with schizophrenia contend with is a 'double loss' – first, a life derailed by schizophrenia, and second, forfeiting the typical dream of success in the new land.

Environment

This category is broadly defined but includes factors that interact with each other, such as location (urban or rural, industrialized or developing region), discrimination and socioeconomic status (poverty, housing and food insecurity). HOPES is a useful mnemonic to assess social and environmental factors in each individual (Figure 3.2). We will discuss these factors when considering the issue of who is at risk for schizophrenia, in Chapter 17.

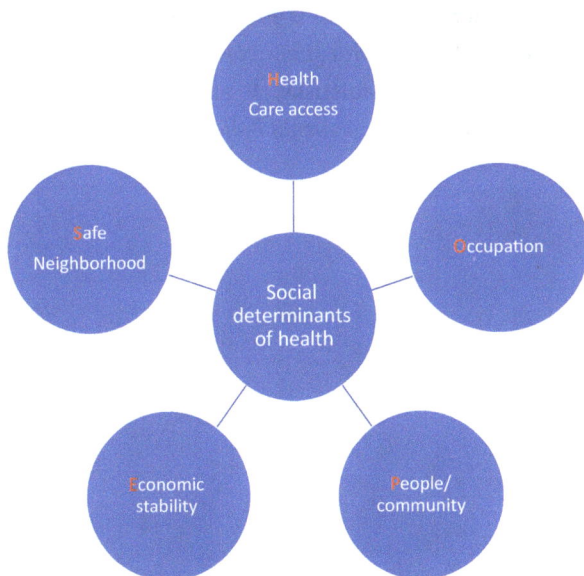

Figure 3.2 Social determinants of health (HOPES).

Summary

- Apart from the illness itself, there are biological, environmental and cultural factors that modify the clinical presentation (and long-term outcome).
- Biological factors include sex, race, age and age of onset of illness.
- Environmental factors include, among others, socioeconomic status, social supports, migration, health-care access, neighborhood safety, and co-morbid psychiatric and medical conditions.
- There is cultural diversity among patients. Culture has powerful effects on illness presentation and illness perception, and it affects relationships with health providers; attention needs to be paid to cultural issues early in assessment and treatment to maximize care of patients.

References

Jester, D. J., Thomas, M. L., Sturm, E. T., Harvey, P. D., Keshavan, M., Davis, B. J., Saxena, S., Tampi, R., Leutwyler, H., Compton, M. T., Palmer, B. W., & Jeste, D. V. (2023). Review of major social determinants of health in schizophrenia-spectrum psychotic disorders: I. Clinical outcomes. *Schizophrenia Bulletin, 49*(4), 837–850.

Robins, L. N., & Regier, D. A. (Eds). (1991). *Psychiatric disorders in America: The epidemiologic catchment area study.* New York: Free Press.

Sartorius, N., Shapiro, R., & Jablensky, A. (1974). The international pilot study of schizophrenia. *Schizophrenia Bulletin, 1*(11), 21–34.

chapter 4

Schizophrenia, spirituality and religion

Religious affiliation and private faith can be important dimensions of a person's life. Defining terms like religion, faith or spirituality is not easy, because these concepts cross many boundaries of human activity. Below are simple, hopefully useful definitions. However, regardless of the formal label that one uses (*I'm Buddhist, I'm Roman Catholic, I'm Muslim*, etc.), it is important to ask the patient or the family what *they* hold to be religious or spiritual.

Religion is the belief in the supernatural, sacred or divine, and the moral codes, practices, values and institutions associated with such belief. Or we might say that religion is a belief in spiritual beings. But most understand religion to mean organized religion, for example, Buddhism, Christianity, Hinduism, Islam and Judaism.

Faith refers to relational aspects of religion. Among its many meanings are loyalty to a religion or religious community or its tenets, commitment to a relationship with God and belief in the existence of God.

Spirituality, often used interchangeably with religion, may or may not include belief in a personal god and in supernatural beings and powers, as in religion, but emphasizes experience at a personal level, as in faith. Spirituality can mean a feeling of connectedness, that life has purpose, and that these perspectives can facilitate personal development.

DOI: 10.4324/9781315152806-4

For those individuals who have had some sort of religious upbringing, personal development determines whether they go on to practice that religion, transform their beliefs or leave behind religion or faith. It is important to find out the patient's religious practices, because the superimposition of a psychotic disorder on pre-existing beliefs can lead to a complicated set of interactions that need to be sorted out.

Religion and psychosis

Belief in the supernatural (good or evil) is common among people all over the world, and therefore it is no surprise that religious themes are present in psychotic phenomena, as are other elements of culture. Religious themes in the context of psychosis include belief in personal persecution by the devil or equivalent; special messages from, or direct communication with, God; special tasks assigned by the divine; God's voice; and becoming God or one of the supernatural beings. These presentations, although recounted in many texts and religious traditions, would not be considered the norm by most adherents of organized religion. On the other hand, in many parts of the world there are traditions that are accepting of all of the above. This, however, does not negate the utility of the definition of a delusion as a fixed, false belief that is *at odds with the community's cultural and religious beliefs*.

When assessing patients presenting with religious delusions, however, it is important not to reflexively attribute these beliefs to psychosis, but to ascertain the cultural context (Table 4.1). If one is not familiar with the cultural background of the patient, it is the clinician's responsibility to find out. Good sources of information include family members, clergy, religious organizations or academics specializing in religious studies.

It is equally important not to assume that all religious expressions in an individual with schizophrenia are pathological and should become the target of treatment! Sometimes a resurgence of faith with the onset of illness can be beneficial. Faith can help allay fears and even bring the patient into the orbit of a church or temple community, widening his or her social network.

Previously held religious beliefs can also become the focus of delusions or hallucinations. It can become difficult to distinguish pathological from normal beliefs under these circumstances. Generally, pathological religious expressions recede with treatment.

Faith can have protective effects. The risk of suicide is lower in patients who have strong belief in traditions forbidding suicide. Substance abuse is likewise decreased because many religions have clear sanctions against intoxicating substances. Prayer can offer a way to cope with all sorts of distress, including hallucinations and delusions.

Table 4.1 Distinguishing normal and pathological religious experiences

	Normative religious beliefs	Pathological religiosity
Phenomenology	Consistent with recognized traditions	May or may not be consistent with traditions
Other indicators of psychiatric disturbance	Absent	Present
Mystical or ecstatic experiences	Persons able to revert to reality	Usually a component of psychotic experience, thus unable to control experience
Insight	Generally persons have insight and understand that others may not share their views	Persons lack insight
Time course	Generally long-lasting	Religious delusions may recede with treatment
Lifestyle	Consistent with personal growth	Not necessarily consistent with personal growth

Religion and the clinician

A clinician's religious beliefs and practices, or lack thereof, can factor into the quality of assessment and therapeutic engagement with his or her patient in this domain. Clinicians must seek supervision in situations where they feel uninformed or conflicted in their care of patients for whom religious traditions play an important role in their illness or recovery. Further, the clinician must respect the patient's need for spiritual succor and not proselytize. It is also important not to 'pathologize' every form of religious expression in patients, lest we deny them opportunities for the genuine uplift and comfort that can be derived from religion or spirituality.

The *Diagnostic and Statistical Manual of Mental Disorders* (DSM-5) provides a framework for evaluating spiritual and cultural aspects as part of a psychiatric assessment. The DSM-5 cultural formulation includes cultural identity, cultural conceptualizations of distress (cultural explanations of the individual's illness), psychosocial stressors and cultural features of vulnerability and resilience (cultural factors related to psychosocial environment and functioning), cultural features (elements) of the relationship between the individual and the clinician and an overall cultural assessment (for diagnosis and care).

In order to be sensitive to patients' concerns about religion or faith, it is not necessary to become an expert on all the existing religions and traditions. It is only necessary that the clinician show interest in these matters, as reflected in the nature of questions they ask (*What kinds of religious belief were you brought up with? What are your thoughts about it now? Do you talk to anyone about your religion?*).

Summary

- Religion, faith and spirituality are important dimensions of quality of life.
- Psychosis and religious beliefs have complex interactions.
- Religious delusions are common, primarily persecutory and grandiose delusions.
- Ascertain the cultural context when assessing patients with religious delusions.
- Do not assume that all religious expressions are pathological.
- Belief can provide comfort and coping skills, be protective (from suicide or substance abuse), and widen the social network. On the other hand, religious delusions can be harmful by provoking violence and suicide and inducing non-adherence to treatment.

chapter 5

Putting together the (clinical) pieces

Steps in diagnosis of schizophrenia

Once sufficient current and past psychiatric and medical history has been gathered and a thorough mental-status examination conducted, these pieces of information have to be put together to arrive at a 'working diagnosis'. This is the first step in managing the patient's illness.

It is tempting to assign a diagnosis of schizophrenia, or another diagnosis associated with psychosis, when it appears patently obvious based on the history and mental-status exam. In spite of such certitude, it is prudent to consider other possible explanations (see Figure 5.1). There can be serious consequences if a 'short-cut' is taken in the diagnostic process, such as:

- missing a diagnosis that is managed differently from a primary psychosis
- assigning a diagnosis prematurely, such as schizophrenia, which can have negative psychological effects on the individual and family
- treating with medications that have potentially serious side effects, some possibly irreversible

A woman, aged 30 years, has been experiencing delusions of persecution and grandeur for nine months along with decreased need for sleep and mood fluctuations. Recently she

How would you proceed in order to arrive at a working diagnosis?

DOI: 10.4324/9781315152806-5

has been alternating between abusing cocaine and alcohol. She comes to the clinic because of recent-onset auditory hallucinations. She reports that six months ago she had an automobile accident while intoxicated, requiring hospitalization.

The algorithm shown in Figure 5.1 is a useful process that is utilized to arrive at diagnosis of schizophrenia or another psychotic disorder. The reasons to exercise care in the diagnostic process are manifold, including missing a diagnosis that is treated differently, labeling an individual with a condition that is stigmatizing and the emotional trauma that a patient and his or her family will have to endure.

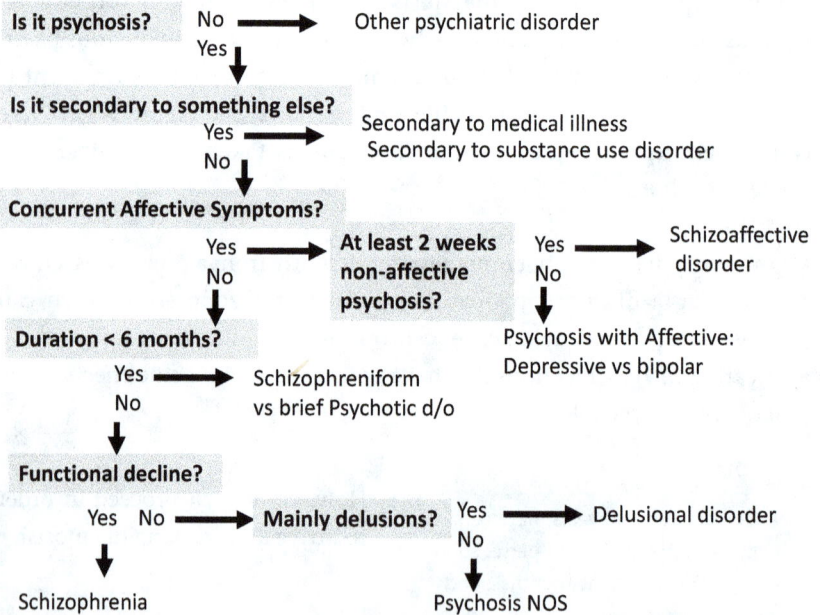

Is it psychosis? No ⟶ Other psychiatric disorder
Yes ↓

Is it secondary to something else?
Yes ⟶ Secondary to medical illness
Secondary to substance use disorder
No ↓

Concurrent Affective Symptoms?
Yes ⟶ **At least 2 weeks non-affective psychosis?** Yes ⟶ Schizoaffective disorder
No ↓ No ↓

Psychosis with Affective:
Depressive vs bipolar

Duration < 6 months?
Yes ⟶ Schizophreniform vs brief Psychotic d/o
No ↓

Functional decline?
Yes No ⟶ **Mainly delusions?** Yes ⟶ Delusional disorder
↓ No ↓

Schizophrenia Psychosis NOS

Figure 5.1 A quick algorithm for DSM-5 differential diagnosis of psychoses.

Could the psychosis be due to a medical condition?

As with elevated body temperature, there are many causes of psychosis, because psychosis is one expression of abnormal brain function. The causes can be broadly categorized according to Table 5.1.

Table 5.1 Differential diagnosis of schizophrenia (TACTICS MDS USE)

Category	Causes (examples)	Investigations
Trauma	Head injury	CT/MRI
Autoimmune	Lupus, NMDA encephalopathy	Antibody titers
Congenital	Velocardiofacial syndrome	Karyotyping
Toxic	Cocaine, amphetamine, PCP, lead	Urine/blood toxic screen
Iatrogenic	Steroids, antimalarials	Urine/blood toxic screen
Cerebrovascular	Stroke	CT/MRI
Space-occupying lesions	Cerebral tumors	CT/MRI
Metabolic	Wilson's disease	Serum copper, caeruloplasmin
Dietary	Pellagra, B12 deficiency	B12, folate levels
Sepsis	Neurosyphillis, HIV	RPR, HIV, LP
Unknown/ degenerative/ demyelinating	Frontotemporal dementia, Huntington's disease, Multiple sclerosis	MRI/PET imaging
Seizure disorder	Temporal lobe epilepsy	EEG
Endocrine	Hyperthyroidism, hypothyroidism, hyperparathyroidism	Thyroid/parathyroid Hormone, calcium levels

The DSM-5 diagnosis that is assigned for psychosis associated with a medical condition is called **psychotic disorder due to a general medical condition.**

If a medical condition is suspected, then thorough and expeditious investigation should be pursued. A medical history and examination at the beginning are critical to rule out potentially reversible causes of schizophrenia-like symptoms (Keshavan & Kaneko, 2013). Laboratory studies vary depending on illness history and physical findings, but all 'first-episode' psychotic patients should probably receive a urine drug screen, complete blood count and measurement of electrolyte levels including calcium, renal, liver and thyroid function tests. A neuropsychological test battery can assist in the diagnosis but is mostly useful to elicit sub-clinical cognitive dysfunction and to establish a baseline for follow-up monitoring. Some clinicians believe all first-episode patients should receive a brain scan and an electroencephalogram. However, some researchers have argued that routine endocrine, electroencephalogram and neuroimaging screening tests are not cost-effective. The choice of assessments should be determined by the probability of detection of abnormalities (especially when there is an atypical presentation of the symptoms), cost, invasiveness and predicted value. Routine use of expensive, invasive investigations should be avoided.

Could the psychosis be due to substance use?

Since substance use (alcohol and illicit drugs) is very common, it needs to be ruled out carefully in every instance of psychosis, even when another obvious explanation for psychosis is available. Substance use can precipitate or cause psychosis and worsen pre-existing psychosis. Substances that can induce psychosis include:

- Alcohol
- Anxiolytics (e.g. diazepam)
- Cannabis
- Cocaine
- Hallucinogens (e.g. LSD)
- Hypnotics
- Inhalants
- Opioids
- PCP and ketamine
- Sedatives
- Stimulants

Table 5.2 Clinical features that may distinguish cannabis-induced psychotic disorders from primary psychotic disorders

	Cannabis-induced psychosis	Primary psychotic disorder
Urine toxicology	Consistently positive for cannabis	Sometimes may be positive
Cannabis history	Cannabis use/escalation Temporally related to psychosis onset	No clear temporal relation between cannabis use and psychosis onset
Course of symptoms	Psychosis subsides with abstinence from cannabis	Psychosis persists despite cannabis non-use
Hallucinations	Tend to be visual/multimodal	Predominantly verbal or auditory
Thought disorder	Uncommon	Common
Insight and cognition	Relatively preserved	Impaired

The DSM-IV diagnosis assigned for psychosis associated with substance abuse or dependence is called **substance-induced psychotic disorder.** Additional DSM diagnoses for substance abuse or dependence would also be assigned.

With the increasing liberalization of cannabis use, cannabis-related psychosis has become an important challenge for differential diagnosis. Table 5.2 provides some tips on how to distinguish between cannabis-related psychosis and a primary psychotic disorder such as schizophrenia. These differences are useful but can be unreliable, and the clinician should keep an open mind and revise the diagnosis if the clinical picture evolves during follow-up.

Could this be a mood disorder with psychotic features?

Mood disorders can be associated with psychosis. This is generally established by determining first whether the criteria are met for one of the mood

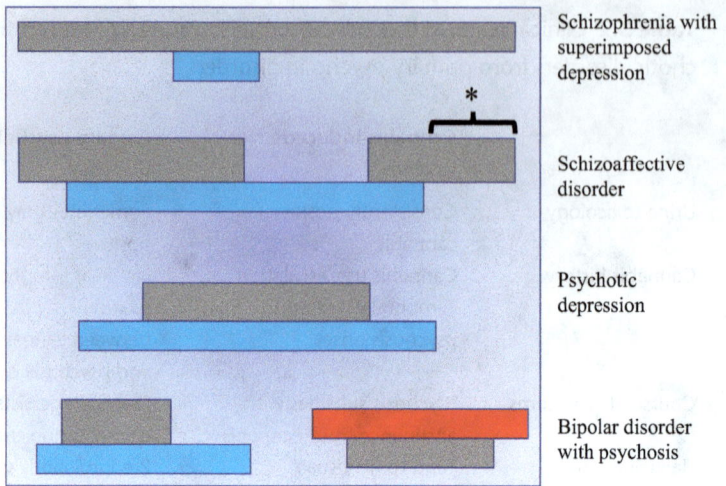

Blue: depression; red: mania; gray: psychosis. * at least 2 weeks of non-affective psychosis needed.

Figure 5.2 Diagnosing psychosis and affective disorders.

disorders and whether the psychosis is present only in the context of the mood disorder. In the DSM-5, mood disorders with psychotic features are major depressive disorder, severe with psychotic features; bipolar I disorder, severe with psychotic features; bipolar II disorder, severe with psychotic features.

Distinguishing affective, schizoaffective and non-affective psychotic disorders can be challenging. A careful history of the chronological relationship between affective and psychotic features can clarify the diagnosis. Figure 5.2 provides a useful way for clinicians to think about the differential diagnosis of psychosis and mood disorders.

Likelihood of a primary psychotic disorder

The primary psychotic disorders, other than schizophrenia, are shown in Table 5.2.

If the above clinical pathway has gotten you this far, it is likely that the condition in question is schizophrenia. However, before proceeding to assign an individual a diagnosis of schizophrenia, one should review the current DSM and ICD criteria as given in Figure 5.3.

Table 5.3 Psychotic disorders

Brief psychotic disorder	Characterized by short-lived psychotic symptoms, typically less than one month, and frequently in relation to a significant psychosocial stressor. The term 'reactive psychosis' has been used in the literature to describe such cases
Schizophreniform disorder	Schizophrenia-like symptoms of acute onset, perplexity or other confusion as part of the clinical picture, relatively intact affect and short duration
Schizoaffective disorder	According to the DSM-5, the diagnostic criteria for schizoaffective disorder are: a) the presence of major depressive or manic episode concurrent with meeting the diagnostic criteria for the active phase of schizophrenia; b) psychotic symptoms for at least two weeks in the absence of prominent affective symptoms during the same episode of illness; and c) the mood-disorder symptoms must be present for a substantial portion of the overall duration of the active and residual periods of the illness. The schizophrenic and affective symptoms can appear simultaneously or in an alternating manner
Delusional disorder	The presence of non-bizarre delusions, that is, delusions involving plausible situations, occurring for at least one month. The absence of prominent hallucinations. Patients with delusional disorder do not have marked impairment in functioning and do not manifest obviously odd or bizarre behavior. There are several types of delusional disorder as per DSM-5, classified on the basis of the content of delusions. These include persecutory, jealous, erotomanic and somatic, as well as mixed types of delusional disorder
Shared psychotic disorder	Also called *folie à deux*, characterized by simultaneous occurrence of psychotic symptoms in two or more individuals. It is a rare psychiatric disorder. There are at least three types of this condition: *Folie imposé*, characterized by the psychotic symptoms imposed by an individual who has a primary psychotic disorder (the dominant partner) on a submissive, suggestible and overly dependent relative who lives in close proximity to the person.

Table 5.3 Continued

	Folie simultanée, characterized by the simultaneous onset of similar psychotic symptoms in two closely related individuals who have a close-knit relationship. *Folie communiquée*, in which one dominant individual induces additional delusions in an individual who already has some psychotic symptoms. *Folie induite*, in which a patient with psychosis adopts another patient's delusion
Culture-bound psychotic disorder	Psychotic syndromes with unique clinical features have been described in a variety of cultures. While the form of symptoms in such syndromes generally conforms to one or another DSM-5 diagnostic category, the content of phenomena such as hallucinations, delusions or unusual behaviors is strongly influenced by culture

Commonly used criteria for the diagnosis of schizophrenia

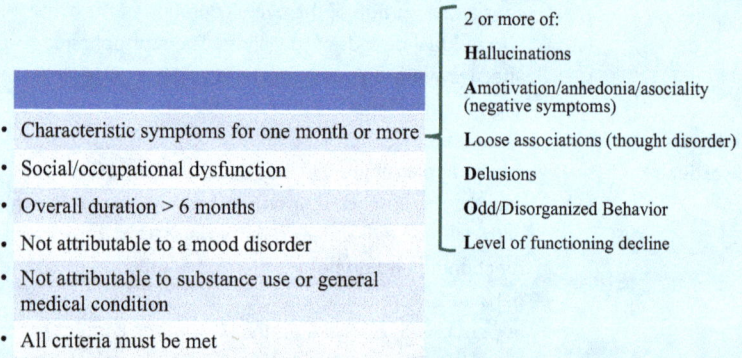

- Characteristic symptoms for one month or more
- Social/occupational dysfunction
- Overall duration > 6 months
- Not attributable to a mood disorder
- Not attributable to substance use or general medical condition
- All criteria must be met

2 or more of:

Hallucinations

Amotivation/anhedonia/asociality (negative symptoms)

Loose associations (thought disorder)

Delusions

Odd/Disorganized Behavior

Level of functioning decline

Figure 5.3 DSM-5 criteria for schizophrenia (note the HALDOL mnemonic).

The DSM-5 is published by the American Psychiatric Press, USA. For the diagnosis of schizophrenia, the DSM requires the presence of at least two of the following symptoms (at least one of which should be 1, 2 or 3) for at least one month:

1. Delusions
2. Hallucinations
3. Disorganized speech
4. Disorganized or catatonic behavior
5. Negative symptoms

Additional criteria include the presence of significant decline in (or failure to achieve adequate functioning in) one or more areas of functioning (work, interpersonal relations or self-care) for a minimum of six months, and the exclusion of schizoaffective disorder and mood disorder with psychotic features. Further, it must be established that the psychosis is not due to the direct physiological effects of a substance (alcohol, drugs of abuse or medications) or a medical condition. Subtyping of schizophrenia has been dropped from DSM-5 because of lack of reliability and limited clinical utility.

ICD-11

The ICD was developed by the World Health Organization, and the latest version, ICD-11 (Reed et al., 2019), began to be implemented in early 2022. The diagnosis of schizophrenia requires the presence, for at least one month, of at least two well-defined symptoms from the following group:

Persistent hallucinations in any modality

Disturbance in thought processing (derailment, irrelevant speech, neologisms)

Catatonic behavior

Negative symptoms

Significant and consistent changes in behavior (e.g., loss of interest, social withdrawal)

However, schizophrenia should not be diagnosed in the presence of extensive depressive or manic symptoms (unless the psychosis preceded the mood symptoms), or in the presence of overt brain disease or states of drug intoxication or withdrawal.

References

Diagnostic and statistical manual of mental disorders. (2022). *Text revision (DSM-5-TR)* (5th ed.). American Psychiatric Association Publishing.

Keshavan, M. S., & Kaneko, Y. (2013, February). Secondary psychoses: An update. *World Psychiatry, 12*(1), 4–15.

Reed, G. M., First, M. B., Kogan, C. S., Hyman, S. E., Gureje, O., Gaebel, W., Maj, M., Stein, D. J., Maercker, A., Tyrer, P., Claudino, A., Garralda, E., Salvador-Carulla, L., Ray, R., Saunders, J. B., Dua, T., Poznyak, V., Medina-Mora, M. E., Pike, K. M., . . . Saxena, S. (2019, February). Innovations and changes in the ICD-11 classification of mental, behavioural and neurodevelopmental disorders. *World Psychiatry, 18*(1), 3–19.

chapter 6

Talking to patients and families

The foremost goal for communication between clinicians, patients and families is the facilitation and strengthening of the therapeutic alliance. This bond can help patients and families accept and deal with illness, improve treatment adherence and manage crises effectively.

Communication with patients and families often begins on a negative note, commonly when a diagnosis of schizophrenia has been reached and needs to be conveyed to them. Giving bad news to patients and their families is one of the most onerous tasks for clinicians. Talking to them about schizophrenia is no different, particularly at the time of initial diagnostic assessment. Frequently it is complicated by denial on the part of patient and family.

Reluctance to accept the presence of the illness may be due to:

- fear of stigma
- fear of loss of self-efficacy
- lack of knowledge
- lack of insight
- fear of retaliation by patient or family members

Talking to patients about your assessment

The ability to communicate your findings depends a lot on the severity of the patient's delusions or thought disorder. Patients who are severely ill may

DOI: 10.4324/9781315152806-6

not be able to follow your presentation, and it is rarely effective to use a direct approach, such as:

I think you have paranoia. We usually see this in schizophrenia . . .

A better approach might be:

You clearly are having difficulties with . . . [symptoms that patient complains about], and I'd like to work with you to help you feel better and also try to figure out what's going on.

It seems that you are/were having symptoms such as hearing voices. What you are experiencing appears to be consistent with a condition called psychosis. Many conditions can cause psychosis, including mood disorders and schizophrenia. Have you heard about schizophrenia?

Given that a critical decision-point in early engagement of psychotic disorders is diagnosis, having conversations about diagnoses with patients and families is critically important. However, there currently are no clear guidelines for when and how to disclose a diagnosis of a psychotic disorder. Discussing the diagnosis and outlook about the illness with patients requires considerable experience and skill, and is not often part of routine psychiatric training. The INSPIRES (individualizing, normalizing, person-centered, information-accurate, reassuring, empowering and outlining next steps) mnemonic (Table 6.1) may be of help to clinicians in developing an approach to sharing the diagnosis while working with patients with psychotic disorders and their families (Keshavan et al., 2022).

Table 6.1 INSPIRES: an approach to sharing a diagnosis

Individualized
Normalizing and non-stigmatizing
Setting-specific
Person-centered
Reassuring
Empathic and empowering
Strategy and next steps

Talking to patients about treatment

Since antipsychotic drugs are the mainstay of treatment of psychosis, they tend to be emphasized during the early course of the illness. Talking to patients about antipsychotic drugs should be done with the same optimistic stance as one would with any highly treatable condition, particularly in the early illness course, because the rates of resolution of the illness are very high with proper treatment.

Patients should be provided with as much detail about their treatment as is tolerable to them. If psychosis is interfering with their ability to be a partner in their treatment, then the clinician should continue to engage in a positive therapeutic stance. When the severity of psychosis decreases and the patient becomes more able to discuss treatment, it should be with a long-term view in mind: that treatment is a means to preventing relapses and 'getting back on track'. Useful resources to provide patients and families for mental health and treatment information include NIMH, SMI Advisor and the National Alliance on Mental Illness. Ken Duckworth's recent book (2022) on mental-health disorders is a valuable reference for patients and families. A list of useful resources is appended at the end of this book.

Talking to families

Generally, the family is the first to notice changes in the patient and may even have been involved in bringing the patient to the hospital or clinic. Nevertheless, the same sensitivity is needed. Families, like patients, are also dealing with the distress of a relative who is acting abnormally (incomprehensibly).

Families respond to a relative's illness in their own unique ways, but typically early responses are characterized by increased involvement and concern, whereas, with progression of illness, late responses can include increased criticism. Both sets of responses, if immoderate, can have negative consequences for the patient (Figure 6.1).

All families need reassurance regarding:

- thoroughness of the clinical assessment
- availability of effective treatment

- being informed and consulted about the care of their relative ('kept in the loop')
- that there are others in the same situation ('you're not alone')
- hope

Statements that don't work:

- *Is anyone in the family schizophrenic? Yes, well that explains it.*
- *Did John have a difficult birth or was he neglected?*

Statements that can be helpful:

- *What has it been like for you all with what John's been going through?*
- *What would be helpful to cope with his illness?*

Families often are integral to the care of patients and should be involved from the beginning and offered support. Schizophrenia is an illness that strikes young adults, who are likely dependent on their families, and this dependency increases further with illness onset.

It is very helpful to provide families with the contact telephone numbers of the treatment team, the hospital emergency number, support groups in the neighborhood and websites with information about schizophrenia.

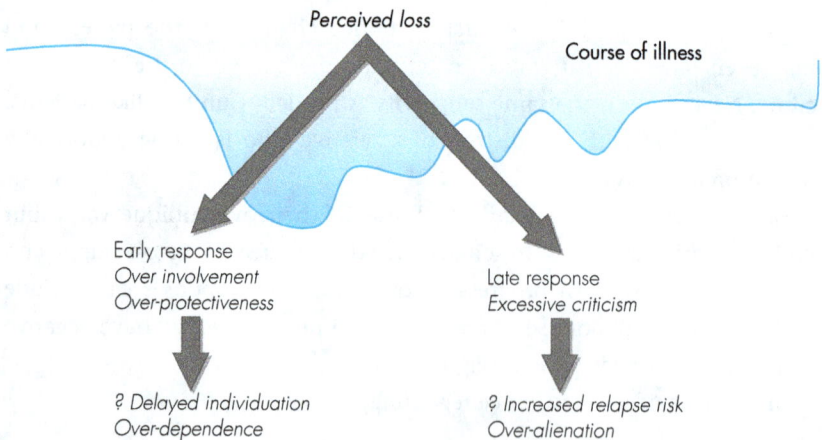

Figure 6.1 Typical family responses to a relative's illness.

Family sessions

It is important to meet with families, with and without the patient, as soon as possible after initiating treatment. The goals of family sessions are to allow the sharing of feelings about what is occurring with their relative, provide them with information about the illness and establish a working alliance with key family members. Involving the family early in the course of treatment can actually help to prevent the patient from alienating him- or herself later. We have found it very useful to insist that initial family sessions include the patient. This largely mitigates any later communication problems between patient and family, between patient and clinician about the family and between clinician and family. During these sessions we encourage openness, sharing of concerns, discussion of the symptoms and distress and development of a collaborative spirit. The need for communication between the clinician and the family, particularly during periods of crisis, should also be discussed.

When meeting with families, be prepared to answer many, and sometimes difficult, questions. Responses to these questions should be honest, but with a non-judgmental and hopeful stance. The types of information that families seek tend to fall into the following categories:

- definition of psychosis
- triggering factors, role of stress
- substance abuse
- denial, compliance issues
- stigma
- impact of illness on family
- prognosis
- dependence and independence issues
- medications, side effects
- difficulties with healthcare system
- depression, suicide

Note about confidentiality

Patients have a right to privacy. The therapeutic alliance is fostered when it is clear that confidentiality will be maintained. Family sessions must be approached with this in mind. A general approach is to ask patients whether there is anything they would not like to share with others. Occasionally, patients will outright forbid contact with family. This is a difficult situation, but these wishes must be respected, although every effort must be made to avoid a split between patient and family. We suggest frequently reviewing the patient's position on this matter because it may alter during treatment. For example, conflicts with family may be due to paranoia, and as it resolves the relations with family may improve. Involving families early in treatment decisions and establishing a spirit of open communication is very helpful in the longer run.

The chief virtue that language can have is clearness, and nothing detracts from it so much as the use of unfamiliar words.

Hippocrates

Language is very important

While presenting a diagnosis, it is important to be cautious about invoking the label 'schizophrenia'. Since its conception over a century ago, the term has been associated with discrimination and stigma. It is often misunderstood (confused with split personality) and used with a negative connotation. For this reason, several initiatives around the world have even attempted to replace the term 'schizophrenia' with alternatives such as 'integration disorder'. A recent, large US survey of multiple stake-holders, including patients and family members, supported this view, and the search continues for names that convey a better understanding of the nature of this illness (Mesholam-Gately et al., 2021). In the meantime, it is important to use this term only after a careful and comprehensive assessment that includes efforts to rule out other related conditions. At initial meetings, it is often better to discuss symptoms and appropriate treatments, and to convey the need to obtain more information over time to clarify a diagnosis.

Maintaining hope

There are few good predictive markers in schizophrenia, and the subjective or 'gut feeling' predictions of experienced clinicians can be overly gloomy compared to careful scientific studies. This 'clinician's illusion' arises from the experience of spending more time caring for those who are suffering the worst outcomes. The reality is that outcomes are actually quite variable, and, for the majority of patients, there are many modifiable prognostic factors that can be targets for clinical and social intervention. The HOPE mnemonic (Table 6.2) can be a useful framework to consider while discussing treatment options and outlook with patients and families.

Instilling hope at the outset is critically important, but what happens in practice is often the opposite. Psychologist and researcher Patricia Deegan (2022) recently recounted being told by a psychiatrist when she was a teenager,

> 'You have a disease called schizophrenia. Schizophrenia is a disease that is a lot like diabetes. Just like a diabetic has to take insulin for the rest of their lives, you'll have to take antipsychotic medication for the rest of your life'. He proceeded to tell me that after discharge, my job was to avoid stress and take high dose antipsychotics religiously, in order to slow the progression of the disease. No romance. No school. Just avoid stress.

Deegan adds, 'No one at the time told me boredom and meaninglessness are profoundly stressful'. Of course, hopeful statements need to be offered with honesty and humility.

Very often, outcomes are influenced by factors unknown at the beginning, such as response to treatment, treatment adherence, psychosocial events and circumstances etc. It is important to present possible outcomes as potentially changeable with the appropriate treatments. It is useful to suggest alternative options, such as long-acting injectables and clozapine, early in the course of the illness, so that patients may be willing to consider them later in the event treatment response is unsatisfactory. Developing a partnership in the context of a positive therapeutic alliance is likely to improve outcomes in the early course of psychotic disorders (Frank & Gunderson, 1990). Using a person-centered approach to consider an individual's unique health needs and desired health outcomes is essential for effective care. Finally, empowering patients and families using a shared decision-making approach can improve outcomes.

Table 6.2 HOPE: an approach to discussing prognosis

Hope, honesty and humility
Options to consider now and for later
Partnership: person-centered care
Empowerment

Outcome and course of schizophrenia

An oft-repeated rule of thumb in the schizophrenia literature is that one-third of patients have a recovering, significantly benign course; one-third have a relapsing/remitting course, with some level of functioning preserved over the course of the illness; and one-third have a chronic illness with persistent impairment. Scientific literature provides some assistance in conveying the odds of a particular outcome, and factors that mediate such outcomes, to patients, families and others who need to know.

Questions a **patient and family** may ask when confronted with illness are:
What will happen next?
Will it ever go away?
Why me?

Questions a **health provider** should ask when confronted with illness are:
How can I help now?
How can I help them plan for the future?
How can I help them cope with the question, 'why me?'

BD is a 22-year-old recently diagnosed with schizophrenia. His family wants to know what to expect. BD did very well in school until he experimented with mushrooms a few times, after which he rapidly developed hallucinations and paranoia. He has a very supportive family.

What would you say to the family?

Being male is generally a risk factor for poorer long-term outcome. BD's onset of illness is at the upper age-range for males (late adolescence to early adulthood), which is more favorable than later age at onset. Drug abuse is commonly observed before and during onset of illness, and

What factors are important in determining BD's prognosis?
a) Gender
b) Age
c) Mushroom abuse
d) Performance in school
e) Rapidity of the onset of psychosis

may not specifically be prognostic unless it becomes chronic. Good premorbid school functioning favors a better outcome. Likewise, rapid onset of illness is associated with good outcome. In summary, although BD is male of typical age at onset of illness, he has several factors in favor of a likely good outcome. Further, he has a supportive family which also bodes well for BD.

What are the predictors of outcome in schizophrenia?

This is of importance both in discussing with patients and family members what to expect down the road, and in estimating return to employment, which is needed for most occupational-disability evaluations. Fortunately, a substantial body of evidence exists to guide the clinician in answering this question (Suvisaari et al., 2018). While individual factors have limited predictive value, collectively considering them may have some value in clinical practice. The following factors have been thought to have some predictive value:

Premorbid maladjustment
Resource limitations
Early onset
Delay in treatment, Deficit symptoms
Inadequate treatment
Cognitive impairment
Treatment non-response
Substance abuse

Another facet of outcome in schizophrenia is the trajectory to the long-term outcome. As can be seen in Figure 6.2, there are several pathways that the illness can take during the course of several years. It is difficult to predict a specific illness course early on.

LK has a three-year history of schizophrenia. He had a very good treatment response at first episode of illness, enabling return to full-time school. One year later he relapsed, requiring hospitalization. He returned to school but could manage only one course. He continued to have low motivation, and occasional paranoid thoughts with social interactions. Recently he relapsed again and now requires a group home.

LK is showing evidence for an episodic course, with inter-episode deficits. On the other hand, if LK's course of illness had been examined two years ago, it might have appeared to be episodic, without inter-episode deficits. Thus, the course of illness is best determined retrospectively.

What is LK's course of illness?
a) Single, unremitting episode
b) Episodic, *without* inter-episode deficits
c) Episodic, *with* inter-episode deficits
d) Chronic, deteriorating

Outcome in schizophrenia is variable

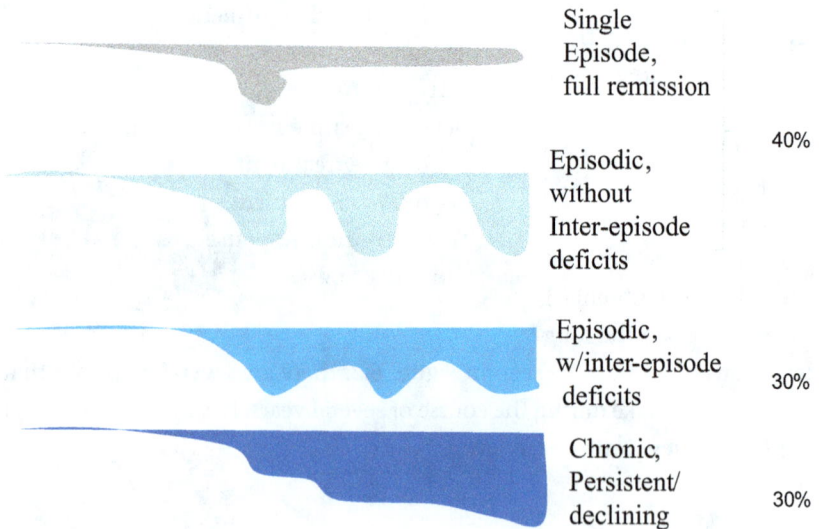

Single Episode, full remission

Episodic, without Inter-episode deficits — 40%

Episodic, w/inter-episode deficits — 30%

Chronic, Persistent/ declining — 30%

Figure 6.2 Outcome trajectories in schizophrenia.

Summary

- Effective communication between clinicians, patients and families facilitates therapeutic alliance, which is essential to good care.
- Talk to patients about treatment with an optimistic stance, particularly since the rates of resolution of first episodes of psychosis are very high.
- Patients should be provided with as much detail about their treatment as is tolerable to them.
- Families, like patients, are also dealing with the stress and trauma of the illness. They also need reassurance that the best is being done for their relative.
- Meet with families as soon as possible, and have at least a few sessions with both patient and family together.
- Be mindful of the confidentiality issues involved in sharing information with family.
- Discussions about prognosis are important. While there are relatively few reliable predictors of long-term outcome, several indicators (PREDICTS) can help organize support and intervention.
- During the early days of the illness, it is important to maintain a hopeful stance with the patient and family. The HOPE acronym summarizes the key principles to consider while discussing the disease outcome with patients and caregivers.

References

Deegan, P. E. (2022, August). I am a person, not an illness. *Schizophrenia Research, 246*, 74.

Duckworth, K. (2022). *You are not alone: The NAMI guide to navigating mental health—with advice from experts and wisdom from real people and families.* NAMI.

Frank, A. F., & Gunderson, J. G. (1990, March). The role of the therapeutic alliance in the treatment of schizophrenia. Relationship to course and outcome. *Archives of General Psychiatry, 47*(3), 228–236.

Keshavan, M. S., Davis, B., FriedMan-Yakoobian, M., & Mesholam-Gately, R. I. (2022, January). What is my diagnosis, Doc? Discussing psychosis diagnosis with patients and families. *Schizophrenia Research, 239*, 92–94.

Mesholam-Gately, R. I., Varca, N., Spitzer, C., Parrish, E. M., Hogan, V., Behnke, S. H., Larson, L., Rosa-Baez, C., Schwirian, N., Stromeyer, C., Williams, M. J., Saks, E. R., & Keshavan, M. S. (2021, December). Are we ready for a name change for schizophrenia? A survey of multiple stake-holders. *Schizophrenia Research, 238,* 152–160.

Suvisaari, J., Mantere, O., Keinänen, J., Mäntylä, T., Rikandi, E., Lindgren, M., Kieseppä, T., & Raij, T. T. (2018, November). Is it possible to predict the future in first-episode psychosis? *Front Psychiatry, 13*(9), 580.

chapter 7

Early intervention and prevention for schizophrenia

The first three to five years after the onset of psychosis should be viewed as a 'critical period' for intervention. Most of the functional decline from these illnesses occurs during this time, and several modifiable adverse prognostic factors emerge in these first few years, including substance misuse, disengagement from treatment and risk for aggression and self-harm (Birchwood et al., 1998).

Despite the common assumption that schizophrenia is invariably associated with poor outcome, systematic studies suggest a more hopeful picture with considerable heterogeneity, and some individuals achieving high levels of recovery. As can be seen in Figure 7.1, patients in groups A and C may have either an excellent or poor recovery, respectively, after their *first* episode. The largest proportion of early course schizophrenia or first-episode psychosis (FEP) patients (group B) have an uneven course with repeated episodes of care and successful reduction of symptoms and distress, often followed by disengagement and relapse (e.g., Srihari et al., 2012). In typical systems of care, this results in a loss of social function, which reaches a stable plateau after about five years. Early-intervention services can improve upon these suboptimal outcomes.

One of the key developments in care for FEP patients has been specialized team-based care – or Coordinated Specialty Care (CSC) – wherein clinicians from several disciplines (e.g., social work, nursing, psychology, psychiatry) coordinate their efforts to provide a comprehensive package of empirically based treatments to young individuals with FEP (and their families) and also address a range of social determinants of outcome (e.g.,

DOI: 10.4324/9781315152806-7

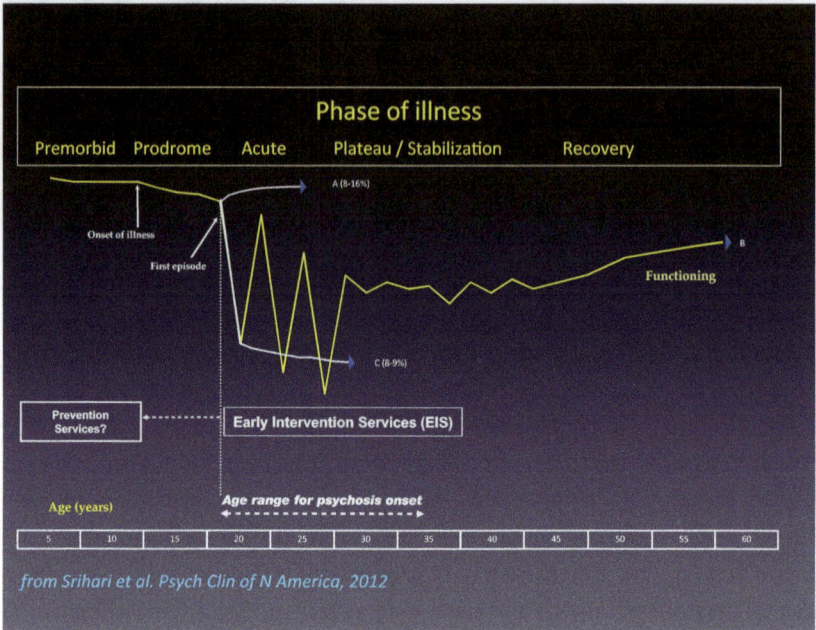

from Srihari et al. Psych Clin of N America, 2012

Figure 7.1 Opportunities for early intervention.

housing, employment, education, access to community resources). CSCs are now a best practice or aspirational standard of care for FEP in the US (Correll et al., 2018).

While CSCs represent an important advance in the *quality* of care, they may have little impact on longer-term outcomes if individuals access them too late. The time from psychosis onset to initiation of treatment, or the Duration of Untreated Psychosis (DUP), is an important predictor of response to CSC: the longer the DUP, the poorer the outcome. Thus, it is also important for early-intervention services to improve *access* by reducing DUP (Srihari et al., 2016).

Design of early intervention services

Models for delivering early intervention – Early Intervention Services (EIS) – are best conceived of as care pathways with component modules that help

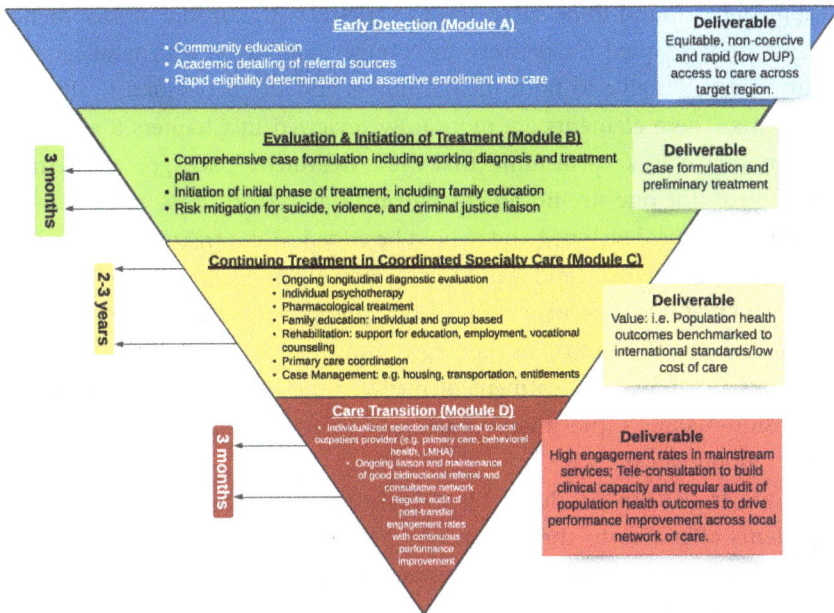

Early Detection (Module A)
- Community education
- Academic detailing of referral sources
- Rapid eligibility determination and assertive enrollment into care

Deliverable
Equitable, non-coercive and rapid (low DUP) access to care across target region.

Evaluation & Initiation of Treatment (Module B)
- Comprehensive case formulation including working diagnosis and treatment plan
- Initiation of initial phase of treatment, including family education
- Risk mitigation for suicide, violence, and criminal justice liaison

Deliverable
Case formulation and preliminary treatment

Continuing Treatment in Coordinated Specialty Care (Module C)
- Ongoing longitudinal diagnostic evaluation
- Individual psychotherapy
- Pharmacological treatment
- Family education: individual and group based
- Rehabilitation: support for education, employment, vocational counseling
- Primary care coordination
- Case Management: e.g. housing, transportation, entitlements

Deliverable
Value: i.e. Population health outcomes benchmarked to international standards/low cost of care

Care Transition (Module D)
- Individualized selection and referral to local outpatient provider (e.g. primary care, behavioral health, LMHA)
- Ongoing liaison and maintenance of good bidirectional referral and consultative network
- Regular audit of post-transfer engagement rates with continuous performance improvement

Deliverable
High engagement rates in mainstream services; Tele-consultation to build clinical capacity and regular audit of population health outcomes to drive performance improvement across local network of care.

3 months

2-3 years

3 months

Figure 7.2 Early Intervention Service care pathway.

organize the efforts of the clinical team, but that are nevertheless experienced as a seamless and coordinated journey to and through care by the patient and family (Figure 7.2).

Early Detection (Module A) includes efforts to reduce DUP and ease the path to accessing the CSC team. These include efforts to minimize interactions with the criminal justice system and involuntary hospitalizations.

Evaluation and Initiation of Treatment (Module B) includes efforts to engage FEP individuals into care. While this is a high-risk period for self-harm, the young individual or family who are disheartened or even angry about their previous experiences of care often do not acknowledge the presence of an illness or do not trust the mental healthcare system. A comprehensive evaluation of these barriers to engagement will assist with building an alliance and initiating elements of treatment that will often need to begin even before a definitive diagnosis and longer-term treatment plan can be developed.

Coordinated Specialty Care, CSC (Module C) builds on the gains made in the prior modules. A variety of pharmacological and psychosocial approaches found to be successful in patients with chronic schizophrenia have been adapted for delivery to younger patients and to families that are relatively naïve to both mental illness and the behavioral healthcare systems. These elements are more fully reviewed in Chapters 8 and 9. It is important to keep in mind that these treatment 'packages' are neither complete nor one-size-fits-all (Keshavan et al., 2022). New interventions continue to be developed and should be added to the treatment repertoire as emerging evidence and feasibility support their use (for example, cognitive interventions). Moreover, it is likely that patients will choose different elements over the course of their care, and this selective utilization of the various psychosocial treatment elements should be welcomed as shared decision-making rather than condemned as evidence of deviation from a rigid model of care.

Care transition (Module D) is relevant for most EIS that must graduate patients after two to three years of care because of resource constraints. Thus, handoff to outpatient services must be done in an informed and gradual manner, with a set of individualized recommendations offered to the new care team.

Earl(ier) intervention and prevention

We now know that schizophrenia spectrum disorders represent an end-point or result of interactions between genetic risk and environmental factors. This neurodevelopmental model suggests that the so-called 'first episode' of psychosis is not the beginning but rather the progression or end-point of processes that are poorly understood. Nevertheless, the syndrome (i.e. combination of subjective symptoms and observable signs) of psychosis is currently the only way to reliably determine the presence of an illness. This is also the phase of the illness where we can justify interventions that are based on strong evidence of effectiveness and safety.

What about prevention? This term is best reserved for efforts that seek to reduce the incidence of an illness or delay its onset, rather than to eradicate it. This generally means targeted interventions in those individuals who are not yet ill but may be at risk. This requires great caution so as not to introduce risks without demonstrable overriding benefits. Clearly, a universal psychosis-prevention program, along the lines of seatbelt mandates or smoking bans, cannot be implemented across an entire population. Alternatively, *selective* prevention can target sub-groups known to be at higher risk for poor outcomes (e.g., alcohol-use reduction among pregnant women to prevent fetal harm). For psychotic disorders, a proposal has been made to limit the use, or at least delay the age of first use, of cannabis. This could serve as both a universal (for all adolescents) and selective (for those known to be at higher risk for schizophrenia) prevention. A third kind of prevention is advisable or *indicated* only when there are subtle signs of an incipient illness and an intervention might be able to delay or prevent progression to a diagnosable disorder. Research on interventions in Clinical High Risk (CHR) individuals known to be at higher risk for a future psychotic episode may yield strategies that reduce the risk of a psychosis episode or at least delay its emergence. Cognitive Behavioral Therapy (CBT)-based approaches show some promise in this regard (Srihari & Keshavan, 2022).

Another approach to at-risk individuals is to develop biomarkers – biological or psychosocial – that will provide targets for preventive intervention. A useful analogy is elevated blood pressure, which is often present in asymptomatic individuals. Once the elevated blood pressure is identified, pharmacological and other lifestyle interventions can be instituted, thereby reducing the risk of complications such as stroke and congestive heart failure. Several candidate biomarkers in schizophrenia offer such a future prospect, and when equivalent evidence emerges, prevention services for the early phases of this illness can be implemented (Figure 7.1). Further discussion of specific biomarkers is included in Chapter 19.

Summary

- Psychotic illnesses are distressing, disabling and costly under usual care.
- Outcomes for these 'chronic illnesses of the young' can be substantially improved via Early Intervention Services (EIS).
- Modern EIS should attempt to improve both Access to (reduce DUP and improve experience of pathway to care) and Quality of (provide Coordinated Specialty Care) care.

- Ongoing research may deliver interventions targeting the pre-psychosis or high-risk phase (earlier intervention) and biomarkers that will enable targeting of the premorbid phase (prevention) of these illnesses. Clinicians should consider joining networks of services to enable sharing of lessons for quality improvement and participation in research.

References

Birchwood, M., Todd, P., & Jackson, C. (1998). Early intervention in psychosis. The critical period hypothesis. *British Journal of Psychiatry*, *172*(33), 53–59.

Correll, C. U., Galling, B., Pawar, A., Krivko, A., Bonetto, C., Ruggeri, M., Craig, T. J., Nordentoft, M., Srihari, V. H., Guloksuz, S., Hui, C. L. M., Chen, E. Y. H., Valencia, M., Juarez, F., Robinson, D. G., Schooler, N. R., Brunette, M. F., Mueser, K. T., Rosenheck, R. A., . . . Kane, J. M. (2018). Comparison of early intervention services vs treatment as usual for early-phase psychosis. *JAMA Psychiatry*. Published online May 2, 2018.

Keshavan, M. S., Ongur, D., & Srihari, V. H. (2022). Toward an expanded and personalized approach to coordinated specialty care in early course psychoses. *Schizophrenia Research*, *241*, 119–121.

Srihari, V. H., Jani, A., & Gray, M. (2016). Early Intervention for psychotic disorders: Building population health systems. *JAMA Psychiatry*, *73*(2), 1–3.

Srihari, V. H., & Keshavan, M. S. (2022). Early intervention services for schizophrenia: Looking back and looking ahead. *Schizophrenia Bulletin*, *48*(3), 544–550.

Srihari, V. H., Shah, J., & Keshavan, M. S. (2012). Is early intervention for psychosis feasible and effective? *Psychiatric Clinics of North America*, *35*, 613–631.

chapter 8

Managing symptoms and preventing relapse

Pharmacological approach

The treatment of schizophrenia was revolutionized in 1952 with the discovery of chlorpromazine as the first effective pharmacological antipsychotic. In the intervening several decades, numerous antipsychotic agents have come to market, offering patients more options to enable either improved response or reduced side effects.

What are antipsychotic agents?

These are a diverse group of drugs used to treat the psychosis syndrome. These drugs do not treat all of the broad range of impairments associated with schizophrenia, but are quite effective at targeting the positive symptoms of psychosis, regardless of cause. Antipsychotic drugs (APDs) used to be referred to as major tranquilizers (inducing calm) or neuroleptics (from *lepsis*, to hold down). These medications can also help manage the symptoms of depression and bipolar disorder, and several have been approved by the FDA as mood stabilizers. This has led to the proposal to replace the potentially stigmatizing and confusing label 'antipsychotics' with one derived from pharmacological properties (e.g., dopamine antagonists, dopamine serotonin antagonists, dopamine partial agonists, etc.). This neuroscience-based nomenclature has been developed for a variety of medications used to treat mental illnesses (Zohar et al., 2015).

DOI: 10.4324/9781315152806-8

During the first 30 years after the discovery of chlorpromazine, attention was focused on drugs that blocked the neurotransmitter dopamine. In the intervening years, research shifted to other neurotransmitters, particularly serotonin. Since the late 1980s, the so-called 'second-generation' APDs have emerged as front-runners in the treatment of schizophrenia. Whereas the 'first-generation' APDs are primarily dopamine antagonists, the newer APDs have different mechanisms of action (dopamine and serotonin antagonists, dopamine partial agonists, etc.). You will discover, however, that *typical (first-generation)* and *atypical (second-generation)* labeling reflects the convenience of common usage rather than a rigorous system of classification based on either effectiveness or pharmacologic properties.

Table 8.1 Advantages and disadvantages of APDs

	Advantages	Disadvantages
First-generation APDs, or FGAs (e.g. haloperidol, fluphenazine, thiothixene)	• Effective with positive symptoms • Low risk of metabolic syndrome • Haloperidol useful in delirium, pregnancy	• No effect on negative symptoms • No effect on cognitive deficits • Extrapyramidal syndromes (EPS) • Prolactin elevation
Second-generation APDs, or SGAs (e.g. aripiprazole, clozapine, olanzapine, quetiapine, risperidone, ziprasidone, lurasidone, lurasidone)	• Effective with positive and negative symptoms and cognitive deficits • Low EPS potential[1] • Lesser prolactin elevation[2]	• Weight gain[3] • Increased risk of metabolic syndrome • Expensive

1. Risperidone at higher doses induces EPS with greater frequency.
2. Risperidone tends to increase prolactin levels.
3. Greatest weight-gain is seen with clozapine and olanzapine.

All APDs have a mix of advantages and disadvantages, the salience of which depends on the clinical situation at hand (see Table 8.1).

Starting antipsychotic treatment

The two most common clinical situations that require initiation of APDs are (1) first-episode psychosis and (2) relapse following discontinuation of treatment by the patient. Clinicians may switch APDs at any time during the course of illness in response to intolerable side effects or suboptimal treatment response.

Initiation of APDs for **first-episode psychosis** requires consideration of the clinical presentation, the treatment setting and concerns about specific side effects. There is no clear data that can help choose among these drugs based on efficacy. In general, the choice depends on which side effects one wishes to *avoid* in a given patient (see Table 8.2). Patients at first episode of psychosis are particularly prone to side effects. Therefore, the starting dose should be low, dose increases should be in small increments, and side effects should be addressed quickly, lest the patient become treatment non-adherent. As indicated by our own and others' research, patients at first-episode of psychosis tend to have very good treatment response (>70%).

Table 8.2 Choosing Antipsychotics

Prescribing Goal	Approaches
Avoid extrapyramidal side- effects	Consider SGAs
Avoid weight gain, metabolic side effects	Avoid clozapine, olanzapine and quetiapine
Avoid sedation	Avoid clozapine, olanzapine and quetiapine
Rapid-acting	Haloperidol IM, fluphenazine, risperidone M-Tab, ziprasidone IM, asenapine sublingual
To improve adherence	LAI Haloperidol, fluphenazine, risperidone, paliperidone, olanzapine, aripiprazole
To address treatment resistance	Consider clozapine
Cost considerations	Haloperidol, fluphenazine, risperidone

Previous treatment history must be ascertained before initiating APDs following **discontinuation of treatment** by the patient. In general, an APD that has worked well in the past is likely to be a good first choice. When such information is not available, the choice may be made based on which side effects one wishes to avoid.

Current standards of practice increasingly favor SGAs as first-line treatment, although FGAs still have important roles in the treatment of schizophrenia, particularly in first-episode patients. Table 8.3 presents brief descriptions of common atypical APDs to familiarize you with their usage characteristics; it does *not* provide all the information needed for their use in specific patients. You should refer to pharmacopeias for details about pharmacodynamics, metabolism and side effects of these drugs.

Drug selection

As noted earlier, there is no convincing research data that can help in choosing one APD over another based on efficacy alone, particularly among the atypical APDs. One approach is to choose an APD based on side effects one wishes to *avoid* (Figure 9.1), along with other considerations such as previous treatment response, preference, route and frequency of administration and cost.

Table 8.3 Prescriptive characteristics of some common atypical APDs. Dose ranges listed below are for the treatment of schizophrenia in adults. You can find more specific guidelines for other indications and for other populations at www.fda.gov/drugs and www.drugs.com.

Olanzapine

Trade names	**Zyprexa, Zydis**
Available dosing (mg)	2.5, 5, 7.5, 10, 15, 20; Zydis 5, 10, 15, 20
Starting dose	5–10 mg daily
Usual daily dose	5–20 mg
Maximum daily dose	40 mg
Metabolism	CYP450: 1A2; 2D6

Risperidone

Trade names	**Risperdal, Risperdal Consta**
Available dosing (mg)	0.25, 0.5, 1, 2, 4, 1/ml solution; Consta IM
Starting dose	1–2 mg daily
Usual daily dose	1–4 mg daily
Maximum daily dose	16 mg
Metabolism	CYP450: **2D6**; 3A4

Quetiapine

Trade name	**Seroquel**
Available dosing (mg)	25, 100, 200, 300
Starting dose	100 mg daily
Usual daily dose	400–600 mg
Maximum daily dose	800 mg
Metabolism	CYP450: 2D6; **3A4**

Ziprasidone

Trade name	**Geodon**
Available dosing (mg)	20, 40, 60, 80
Starting dose	20–40 mg daily
Usual daily dose	40 mg
Maximum daily dose	80 mg
Metabolism	CYP450: **3A4**

Aripiprazole

Trade name	**Abilify**
Available dosing (mg)	5, 10, 15, 20, 30
Starting dose	10–15 mg daily
Usual daily dose	10–15 mg
Maximum daily dose	30 mg
Metabolism	CYP450: 2D6, **3A4**; poor 2D6 metabolizers have 60% increased drug exposure

Clozapine

Trade name	**Clozaril**
Available dosing (mg)	12.5, 25, 100
Baseline testing	White blood count (WBC), repeated weekly for six months, then biweekly
Starting dose	12.5–25 mg daily
Usual daily dose	300–600 mg

Table 8.3 Continued

Maximum daily dose	900 mg
Metabolism	CYP450: **1A2; 2D6; 3A4**

Lurasidone

Trade name	**Latuda**
Available dosing (mg)	10, 20, 40, 60, 80
Starting dose	40 mg daily
Usual daily dose	80–160 mg
Maximum daily dose	160 mg
Metabolism	CYP450: **1A2; 2D6; 3A4**

Brexpiprazole

Trade name	**Rexulti**
Available dosing (mg)	0.25, 0.5, 1, 2, 3
Starting dose	0.5 mg daily
Usual daily dose	2–4 mg
Maximum daily dose	4 mg
Metabolism	CYP450: **2D6; 3A4**

Cariprazine

Trade name	**Vraylar**
Available dosing (mg)	1.5, 3, 4.5, 6
Starting dose	1.5 mg daily
Usual daily dose	3 mg
Maximum daily dose	6 mg
Metabolism	CYP450: **2D6; 3A4**

Asenapine

Trade name	**Saphris**
Available dosing (mg)	2.5, 5, 10 (sublingual tablets)
Starting dose	5 mg sublingually daily
Usual daily dose	5 mg sublingually two times a day, if tolerated may increase to 10 mg sublingually two times a day after one week if necessary
Maximum daily dose	20 mg
Metabolism	CYP450: **2D6; 3A4**

Iloperidone

Trade name	**Fanapt**
Available dosing (mg)	1, 2
Starting dose	1 mg twice daily
Usual daily dose	6–12 mg twice daily
Maximum daily dose	12 mg twice daily
Metabolism	CYP450: 2D6; 3A4

Lumateperone

Trade name	**Caplyta**
Available dosing (mg)	10.5, 21, 42
Starting dose	42 mg once daily
Usual daily dose	42 mg
Maximum daily dose	42 mg
Metabolism	CYP450: **3A4**

Drug titration and treatment duration

When initiating treatment, you should almost always **start low, go slow**. The aim of treatment is to arrive at maximal therapeutic benefit using the lowest effective dose while minimizing side effects. This is best achieved with the 'low and slow' approach. It is also important to educate patients about likely side effects, giving them a contact number to call in the event of significant side effects, and promptly address the side effects before they lead to non-adherence. Decreasing the likelihood of side effects will enhance treatment adherence, in turn improving treatment response.

Most patients respond to 300–700 mg chlorpromazine *equivalents* (relative potency of APDs compared to a standard dose of chlorpromazine). Table 8.4 provides chlorpromazine equivalents of common APDs; however, this is not a substitute for careful clinical titration against the response and side effects of individual patients. Also, while Chlorpormazine equivalents are better defined for FGAs and are also useful when switching from FGAs to SGAs, for most SGAs there are now dosing guidelines based on patient studies that can provide a useful range of doses within which response is expected to occur (Table 8.5).

Questions that often arise in the course of medication treatment include:

- *How long should the APD be continued at the dose effective for the acute phase?*
- *How long is treatment continued when symptoms have remitted?*
- *How long is an adequate treatment trial?*
- *Can treatment ever be stopped?*

Patients and families tend to be concerned mostly about the last question. Evidence suggests most patients will need maintenance treatment to prevent relapses. After remission of an acute episode, the same APD and the dose that was effective should be maintained for at least a year and probably longer. Discontinuing treatment at any point increases the risk of relapse. There are rare patients who have one episode of psychosis that remits completely and for whom discontinuing APDs may not worsen outcome. However, this is not predictable in advance, so careful, guided discontinuation should only be attempted for selected patients who are well educated about relapse, are at lower risk (based on one or few prior psychotic episodes) and have a support system that is able to alert them and their prescribers to any re-emergence of symptoms. More research is needed for determining the duration of maintenance after an initial episode of schizophrenia. For now, clinicians should recommend continuous antipsychotic treatment using the best-tolerated antipsychotic at minimum effective maintenance doses (Emsley et al., 2016).

Table 8.4 Chlorpromazine equivalents

Chlorpromazine	100 mg
Haloperidol	2 mg
Fluphenazine	2 mg
Risperidone	2 mg
Olanzapine	5 mg
Quetiapine	75 mg
Ziprasidone	60 mg
Aripiprazole	7.5 mg
Haloperidol decanoate	5 mg every four weeks
Fluphenazine decanoate	10 mg every two weeks

Table 8.5 Olanzapine (1 mg/day) equivalents

Aripiprazole	1.4 mg
Chlorpromazine	38.9 mg
Clozapine	30.6 mg
Haloperidol	0.7 mg
Risperidone	0.4 mg
Ziprasidone	7.9 mg

Derived from Leucht et al. (2015).

Common problems during a psychotic episode

Arousal and agitation

There can be many reasons for an agitated state. Patients with paranoia are fearful and may become aggressive as a means of self-defense. Agitation can also be due to irritability, intoxication, substance abuse and withdrawal states and akathisia (drug-induced restlessness), all of which can be present alongside schizophrenia. The first order of business is safety of patient, caregivers and staff. Non-pharmacological approaches – including stimulus reduction and verbal de-escalation using a calm demeanor – should always be tried before using pharmacological treatments. Short-term benzodiazepines, such as lorazepam or clonazepam, have been found to be very effective in decreasing agitation with relatively few undesirable side effects. An advantage of benzodiazepines is their availability in both oral and parenteral formulations. It is preferable to offer oral preparations before resorting to intramuscular (IM) injections. Rapid acting preparations of APDs (e.g., risperidone M tablets, asenapine sublingual, and IM olanzapine or ziprasidone) can also be used in the treatment of agitation. APDs are associated with significantly more side effects requiring vigilance. Acute agitation may require seclusion and restraints, but only as a last resort.

Insomnia

The quantity, initiation and maintenance of sleep are frequently affected in schizophrenia, particularly during florid states. Lack of adequate sleep can contribute to irritability and exacerbation of psychosis. Some APDs have sedation as an early side effect that can be advantageous in this situation. If insomnia persists, short-term oral benzodiazepines (e.g. temazepam 10–20 mg, clonazepam 1–2 mg) or hypnotics (e.g. zopiclone 7.5 mg or zolpidem 5–10 mg) can be utilized. These drugs should be used sparingly, because of their addictive potential. Chronic insomnia requires systematic evaluation and management. Referral to a sleep-evaluation clinic is appropriate.

Summary

- APDs are a diverse group of drugs used to treat psychotic symptoms, not just schizophrenia.
- First-generation APDs are primarily dopamine-blocking drugs. Second-generation APDs have different mechanisms of action, affecting dopamine and serotonin neurotransmission.
- There are no clear data that can help choose among APDs based on efficacy alone. One approach is to choose an APD based on the side effects one wants to avoid., or dopamine partial agonism.
- When an APD is being restarted, choose an APD that has worked well in the past.
- SGAs are increasingly used as first-line treatment for first-episode patients with schizophrenia.
- *Start low, go slow* when initiating treatment.
- Most patients respond to 300–700 mg chlorpromazine equivalents, but consult current prescribing guideline for usual ranges for each SGA.
- Maintain the effective APD dose for at least a year, and consider guided discontinuation only in carefully selected patients.
- Treatment is likely to be continuous and indefinite for most patients with schizophrenia, but clinicians should use the minimum effective dose of the best-tolerated APD for maintenance treatment.

References

Emsley, R., Kilian, S., & Phahladira, L. (2016, May). How long should antipsychotic treatment be continued after a single episode of schizophrenia? *Current Opinion in Psychiatry, 29*(3), 224–229.

Leucht, S., Samara, M., Heres, S., Patel, M. X., Furukawa, T., Cipriani, A., Geddes, J., & Davis, J. M. (2015, November). Dose equivalents for second-generation antipsychotic drugs: The classical mean dose method. *Schizophrenia Bulletin, 41*(6), 1397–1402.

Zohar, J., Stahl, S., Moller, H. J., Blier, P., Kupfer, D., Yamawaki, S., Uchida, H., Spedding, M., Goodwin, G. M., & Nutt, D. (2015, December). A review of the current nomenclature for psychotropic agents and an introduction to the Neuroscience-based Nomenclature. *European Neuropsychopharmacology, 25*(12), 2318–2325.

Psychosocial approaches to improve symptoms and functional outcomes

While antipsychotic drugs (APDs) are largely effective in controlling the severity of positive symptoms, many patients continue to experience distressing delusions and hallucinations. Even with the newer APDs, improvements in overall disability are limited. Thus, a comprehensive approach to overall management, including individual, group and community-based psychosocial treatments, is critically important. It is easy to forget – because of the initial focus on the pharmacotherapy of positive symptoms – that psychosocial treatments are integral to treating schizophrenia from the outset, not as an afterthought. Just as there have been many advances in pharmacotherapy, there have been recent major advances in a variety of psychosocial treatment modalities (Solmi et al., 2023).

The main forms of psychosocial interventions and their role in managing the therapeutic goals in schizophrenia are listed in Figure 9.1. Table 9.1 outlines some scenarios for your consideration.

Psychoeducation

Psychoeducational approaches increase patients' knowledge of, and insight into, their illness and its treatment, enabling people with schizophrenia to cope in more effective ways, thereby improving prognosis. Several clinical trials have shown that psychoeducation programs reduce relapse, improve symptomatic recovery and enhance psychosocial and family outcomes. To be successful, psychoeducation needs to be timely, repeated as necessary and

DOI: 10.4324/9781315152806-9

Goals

Approaches

- Symptoms

- Family functioning

- Treatment adherence

- Substance misuse

- Cognitive deficits, social skills deficits

- Psychoeducation, supportive therapy
- Cognitive behavior therapy
- Mindfulness based therapies
- Family focused treatments
- Motivational interviewing
- Substance use counseling
- Assertive community treatment, case management
- Meta-cognitive therapies
- Cognitive remediation
- Social skills training

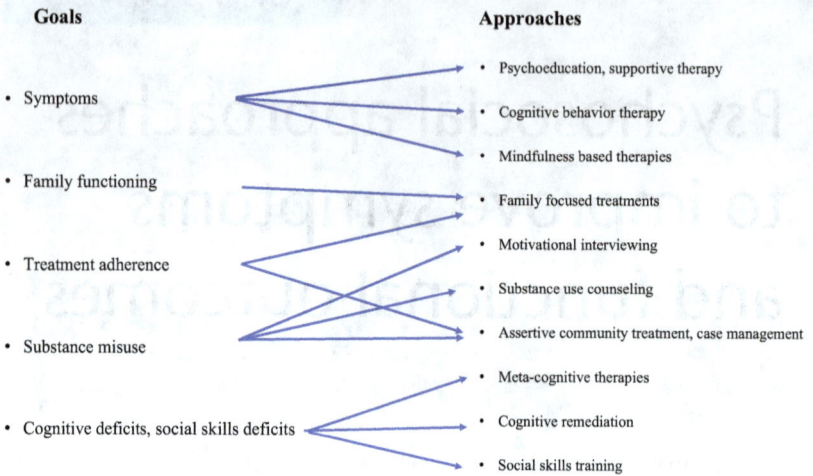

Figure 9.1 Individualized psychotherapy.

Table 9.1 What approach would you choose for the scenario below?

A. The patient is finding it difficult to arrange a variety of appointments for follow-up, groups, pharmacy, job etc.

B. The patient frequently runs out of medications and starts calling the ambulance, worried about imminent relapse.

C. The patient has been admitted to the inpatient service and requires housing that supervises medication administration and follow-up with medical services for diabetes.

D. The patient has been placed with his family after discharge for first episode of schizophrenia. The parents blame themselves for their son's illness. The siblings are increasingly critical because the patient does not do his 'share' of chores at home.

E. The patient has been in partial remission after one year of treatment and now wishes to start a part-time job that primarily involves data entry. He has no means of transportation and has never worked before.

F. After one year of gradually resolving symptoms, the patient returns to her family and discovers that most of her friends are no longer contacting her. She wishes to start making acquaintances, particularly males, but feels unable to do so. She has no way of getting around.

Answers to scenarios in Table 9.1

A. Case management
B. Intensive case management (ICM) or assertive community treatment (ACT)
C. ACT and supported housing
D. Family intervention and psychoeducation
E. Supported employment and ICM
F. Social skills training and case management

tailored to the patient's or family members' cultural and educational background. Individual and group settings, as well as family groups, are effective.

While there are many varieties of psychoeducation, they all embrace a set of core principles that are aimed at maximizing the chances of recovery through education. Our version of psychoeducation has two components (Table 9.1): **TEACH**, which focuses on the process of conveying information; and **I'M SCARED**, which describes the content of the education that addresses the fears that patients and families have about how to cope with the illness and what the future holds for them. The key elements of the program are listed in Table 9.2.

Table 9.2 Psychoeducation principles

TEACH	I'M SCARED
Timely: provide education early	Internal monitoring of mental state & meaning of psychosis
Empower: give as much control as possible to patient/family	
	Medication effects – positive & negative effects
Adapt education to match educational, cultural background	
	Stigma
Continuous education: repeat often; confirm understanding	Coping skills to reduce stress
	Allying with family, friends and clinicians

Table 9.2 Continued

Hopeful: positive; avoid premature labeling/ prognostication	
	Relapse recognition
	Evolving – planning for the future
	Drug abuse prevention

Managing symptoms

In spite of optimal treatment, about a third of patients experience persistent hallucinations and delusions that can be quite distressing. A variety of strategies can be offered to help patients cope and even reduce the severity of hallucinations (Table 9.3) and delusions (Table 9.4).

Table 9.3 ABCs of coping with hallucinations

Arousal reduction	Relaxation and deep breathing exercises
	Blocking ears, closing eyes
	Listening to music
Behavior	Increasing non-social activity
	Reality testing
	Seeking opinions from others
Cognition	Distraction
	Ignoring
	Positive self-talk

Table 9.4 Delusions **BARRED**

Become aware	Increase awareness of delusional thoughts and assumptions
Alternative explanations	Utilize alternative (more neutral) explanations for delusional thought
Record	Monitor and record delusional thoughts
Relaxation techniques	Deep breathing and distraction techniques

| Esteem | Improving self-esteem helps cope with delusions of low worth (often due to derogatory auditory hallucinations) |
| Double book keeping | A mental trick of being able to keep two incongruent ideas in mind without undue distress. For example, believing that one is a millionaire yet living within very limited means |

Cognitive behavioral therapy

Cognitive behavioral therapy (CBT) aims to realign negative or distorted thinking in order to reduce distress. It has been an evolving treatment modality since the 1950s and has been extensively applied in the treatment of depression, anxiety disorders and personality disorders.

Cognitive behavioral therapy focuses on identifying situations and thoughts that are associated with distress, finding acceptable alternative perspectives and then practicing new ways of thinking and behaving outside the therapy session (i.e. homework). CBT is effective in reducing persistent positive symptoms in chronic patients, in preventing relapses, and may even speed recovery in acutely ill patients. CBT also helps the depressive and negative symptoms of schizophrenia. A specialized form of CBT, Cognitive Behavioral Therapy for psychosis (CBTp) has been developed as an individual as well as a group-based intervention (Mander & Kingdon, 2015).

In CBT, symptoms such as delusions and hallucinations are seen as stemming from information-processing biases such as the tendency to overestimate coincidences, jump to conclusions, attribute internal events to external sources and blame others when things are not going well.

Some terms used in CBT

- **Automatic thoughts** come to mind when a particular situation occurs, leading to maladaptive behavior. CBT aims to challenge automatic thoughts
- **Cognitive restructuring** is the process of replacing maladaptive (negative) thought patterns (schemas) with constructive and positive thoughts and beliefs
- **Relaxation techniques** used to relieve stress include biofeedback, meditation and exercise
- **Schemas** are core beliefs or assumptions that serve as filters through which we view the world

Mindfulness-based therapies

Mindfulness refers to a metacognitive process of paying attention to the present moment and detached observation of one's thoughts and feelings. While this approach comes originally from eastern traditions, it has been introduced in the west using a secular approach as a strategy to improve outcomes associated with chronic illnesses. Two approaches that have been used in schizophrenia are mindfulness-based stress reduction and mindfulness-based cognitive therapy. Acceptance-based approaches include dialectical behavior therapy and acceptance and commitment therapy. Emerging literature suggests that these interventions are effective for treatment of people with schizophrenia, although this literature needs to be viewed with caution because of the heterogeneity of results and limited sample sizes (Hodann-Caudevilla et al., 2020),

Improving treatment engagement

Motivational interviewing

Treatment non-adherence is a major concern in the management of schizophrenia (see Chapter 12). There is some evidence that a therapeutic technique known as motivational interviewing (MI) can help to improve treatment adherence in schizophrenia. MI is a counseling technique for motivating behavior change by helping patients to explore and resolve ambivalence. One approach that uses this technique is compliance therapy (CT). Compliance therapy is based on brief motivational interviewing and cognitive therapy techniques. CT has been shown to improve patients' attitudes to drug treatment, insight and treatment adherence and reduce hospital admission rates. Typically, CT involves four to six sessions of 20–60 minutes each.

The ABCs of motivational interviewing

- *Assessment and alliance building.* Review the patient's history; formulate patient's approach to treatment; link medication discontinuation and relapse (ask the patient: *Do you think there is a link between you stopping the medicine and ending back in the hospital?*)

- *Behavior change.* Explore the ambivalence towards treatment; help patient identify benefits and disadvantages
- *Consolidation.* Encouraging self-efficacy; reframing medication as a way to enhance quality of life

Peer support

Peer support, a growing movement, refers to services offered by individuals with lived experience of mental illness to others in similar need. This can offer unique assistance to enhance the patient's acceptance, engagement and response to treatment. In order to become a peer provider, one must transition from being a patient to a provider. Evidence for efficacy of peer support is limited, although patients report subjective benefits; on the other hand, there are few negative consequences to this approach to treatment. Additionally, research on lived experience of psychosis can lead to a better understanding of psychosis, reduced stigma and provision of more person-centered care.

Preventing relapse: family therapy

Family involvement characterized by high expressed emotion (EE: hostility, criticism, overprotection) is associated with higher relapse rates. Family intervention employs educational efforts and behavioral therapy focused on preventing criticism and hostility. If EE cannot be defused, it is prudent to recommend that the patient live in an alternative setting. Family interventions also reduce family burden and improve family well-being. Effective approaches in family intervention include empathic engagement, education, ongoing support, clinical resources during periods of crisis, social network enhancement and problem-solving and communication skills. There is a substantial evidence base for the effectiveness of this approach in preventing relapse (McFarlane, 2016).

Improving functioning

Cognitive training

Cognitive dysfunction, now considered a fundamental feature of schizophrenia affecting 40–95% of individuals, contributes significantly to disability.

Cognitive functions affected in schizophrenia are:

- attention
- working memory (e.g. capacity to keep things in mind long enough for immediate use, such as a phone number)
- learning
- general memory
- forward planning
- concept formation
- initiating action
- self-monitoring

Cognitive training involves three principles (ARC): a) modify the patient's life situation to reduce cognitive demands (adaptation); b) repeated training to harness the brain's own ability to reverse its deficits via neuroplasticity (remediation); and c) use of strategies to 'bypass' some of the cognitive deficits (compensation) (Keshavan et al., 2014). Cognitive remediation strategies vary widely in duration, intensity, method, target of behavioral intervention and clinical status of participants. Using these approaches, improvements have been observed on measures of working memory, emotion perception and executive function. Cognitive enhancement therapy (CET), a form of cognitive remediation developed by researchers at Pittsburgh and Boston, focuses on deficits in cognition and social cognition (the ability to act wisely in social interactions) that are thought to impede social and vocational recovery. Social cognition is acquired during adolescence and early adulthood. CET is designed to facilitate the individual's transition from prepubertal to young-adult style of social cognition. The treatment involves helping the individual to develop a 'gistful' appraisal of interpersonal behavior and novel social contexts.

Social skills training

Verbal and non-verbal skills that aid in communicating with others are required for socialization (the behavior patterns of the culture). These skills include the ability to hold a conversation, make 'small talk', listen actively, use appropriate body language including eye contact, pay attention and express interest. Social skill deficits are a hallmark of schizophrenia. Patients with schizophrenia often develop these deficits after the emergence of the illness, while some have these deficits long before the onset of psychosis. These troublesome deficits are likely due to a combination of positive and negative symptoms as well as cognitive deficits, and can lead to shrinking social networks and feelings of loneliness.

Social skills training (SST) is a well-researched and widely used intervention (Kopelowicz et al., 2006). It seeks to improve psychosocial functioning by helping to improve communication skills needed for interpersonal and vocational goals. Social skills training is based on behavior therapy principles. Complex social skills, such as making friends, are broken down into simpler and smaller steps and then taught using a variety of techniques, including didactic and Socratic instruction, modeling, corrective feedback and homework exercises. SST can be conducted in individual and group sessions. Strategies include assessment of barriers to care, role-playing, social modelling and homework assignments to practice skills in real life situations.

Promoting recovery

Recovery involves addressing a multiplicity of needs which patients with schizophrenia encounter even after symptom control and functional recovery. Multiple social determinants of health can act in concert to yield poor outcomes in schizophrenia (see also chapter 3), despite the best treatment efforts by clinicians, and need to be addressed (Jester et al., 2023). This can be thought of as achieving **HOPE** for patients through the following:

Housing
Occupation

People and networks
Economic independence

Case management and assertive community treatment

Case management is about helping patients negotiate their environment so as to maximize recovery. Treatment of schizophrenia can be a confusing choreography, involving visiting the doctor for follow-up care, obtaining medications, attending groups and rehabilitation activities, arranging transportation for these visits and so forth. Attending to these tasks can be a challenge for patients, even during the recovering phase. Faltering by the patient in attending to different aspects of treatment can increase the risk of relapse. Case management, which includes a wide range of activities such as outreach, crisis intervention, public education and resource management, can be highly effective in maintaining patients in the community and improving outcome.

Assertive community treatment (ACT) is an intensive form of case management which involves social services and rehabilitation delivered by an interdisciplinary mental-health team. Elements of this intervention include staff continuity and continuous responsibility. Staff-to-patient care ratios tend to be high, and frequent, brief visits with patients are typical. This approach is valuable for patients transitioning out of inpatient care who continue to be ill and treatment non-adherent, with a high risk of relapse. ACT is effective in reducing relapse rates and treatment costs in schizophrenia (Scott & Dixon, 1995).

Supported employment and education

Most patients with schizophrenia live in the community, but many are socially isolated, and few have jobs. Conventional approaches to vocational rehabilitation tend not to work well with patients because of the nature of schizophrenia. It is more useful to identify supported worksites that are familiar with the challenges faced by patients with schizophrenia. Jobs that have flexible hours, are relatively stress-free and offer privacy are particularly helpful.

Table 9.5 Principles of supported employment

Incentivized, paid employment is the goal

Inclusion of all patients who want to work
Individual's choice for rapid job search and placement
Integrated employment and health-care team
Individualized support

Supported employment is based on the view that anyone can gain and keep competitive employment and pursue academic goals. It takes the approach of 'place and train', as opposed to the traditional vocational reha- bilitation model of 'train and place'. Supported employment requires assess- ment of goals and skills, rapid job search and assistance with placement in a setting with employers willing to hire patients. Individuals receive support throughout their period of employment (Table 9.5). Supportive employment, along with coordinated clinical care, has been found to increase rates of competitive employment, decrease hospital admissions and improve treat- ment compliance (Drake et al., 2000).

Supported education, like supported employment, provides support for individuals with schizophrenia to achieve academic success using one or more strategies. These include mental-health support on or off the educa- tional site, integrating school or college health services with ongoing men- tal-health care and the use of specialized educational services before the individual moves to integrated classrooms.

In combination with social skills training and/or cognitive remediation, supported employment or supported education may enhance the individu- al's ability to meet the interpersonal demands of the workplace.

Supported housing

Among the many factors that contribute to quality of life, safe and afford- able housing is particularly important. The type of housing a patient requires will depend on his or her capacity to attend to housekeeping chores and general safety. Housing is an evolving 'process', in which patients may initially require a highly supervised group-home setting but over time transition to independent living. Ancillary services, such as mobile case management, crisis intervention and continuous treatment services are often required to enable patients to be managed in the housing of their choice. Patients and clinicians often prefer this approach, since quality of life is usually increased, and length of hospitalizations may also be reduced.

Substance abuse treatment

Twelve-step programs such as Alcoholics Anonymous (AA) and Narcotics Anonymous (NA) are widely used in the treatment of substance-use disorders in schizophrenia, However, they do not always address comorbid disorders in an integrated manner, are sometimes reluctant to include medication treatments and often have somewhat inflexible goals. For these reasons, they may not be effective for many patients unless integrated with other approaches to treatment. Such strategies include family therapy, cognitive behavior therapy, motivational interviewing, lifestyle modifications and social skills training (Mueser & Gingerich, 2013).

Summary
- While antipsychotics are very effective for psychosis, psychosocial treatments are critically important to reduce overall disability.
- Psychoeducational approaches increase patients' knowledge of, and insight into, their illness and its treatment.
- Psychotic and affective symptoms can be improved by utilizing a combination of cognitive behavior therapy and mindfulness-based techniques. Cognitive behavioral therapy (CBT) focuses on identifying situations and thoughts that are associated with distress.
- Cognitive remediation and social skills training involve learning strategies that enhance cognition or improve social skills to address functional impairments common in schizophrenia.

- Addressing social determinants of health, such as housing, occupation, supportive connections with people and economic needs ('HOPE'), is critically important in promoting recovery. Several evidence-based psychosocial approaches, such as supported housing, employment and education, are valuable components of coordinated care for people with schizophrenia.

References

Drake, R. E., Mueser, K. T., Torrey, W. C., Miller, A. L., Lehman, A. F., Bond, G. R., Goldman, H. H., & Leff, H. S. (2000, October). Evidence-based treatment of schizophrenia. *Current Psychiatry Reports, 2*(5), 393–397.

Hodann-Caudevilla, R. M., Díaz-Silveira, C., Burgos-Julián, F. A., & Santed, M. A. (2020, June 30). Mindfulness-based interventions for people with schizophrenia: A systematic review and meta-analysis. *International Journal of Environmental Research and Public Health, 17*(13), 4690.

Jester, D. J., Thomas, M. L., Sturm, E. T., Harvey, P. D., Keshavan, M., Davis, B. J., Saxena, S., Tampi, R., Leutwyler, H., Compton, M. T., Palmer, B. W., & Jeste, D. V. (2023, April 6). Review of major social determinants of health in schizophrenia-spectrum psychotic disorders: I. Clinical outcomes. *Schizophrenia Bulletin, 49*(4), 837–850. https://doi.org/10.1093/schbul/sbad023

Keshavan, M. S., Vinogradov, S., Rumsey, J., Sherrill, J., & Wagner, A. (2014, May). Cognitive training in mental disorders: Update and future directions. *American Journal of Psychiatry, 171*(5), 510–522.

Kopelowicz, A., Liberman, R. P., & Zarate, R. (2006, October). Recent advances in social skills training for schizophrenia. *Schizophrenia Bulletin, 32*(Suppl. 1), S12–S23.

Mander, H., & Kingdon, D. (2015, February 18). The evolution of cognitive-behavioral therapy for psychosis. *Psychology Research and Behavior Management, 8*, 63–69.

McFarlane, W. R. (2016, September). Family interventions for schizophrenia and the psychoses: A review. *Family Process, 55*(3), 460–482.

Mueser, K. T., & Gingerich, S. (2013). Treatment of co-occurring psychotic and substance use disorders. *Social Work in Public Health, 28*(3–4), 424–439.

Scott, J. E., & Dixon, L. B. (1995). Assertive community treatment and case management for schizophrenia. *Schizophrenia Bulletin, 21*(4), 657–668.

Solmi, M., Croatto, G., Piva, G., Rosson, S., Fusar-Poli, P., Rubio, J. M., Carvalho, A. F., Vieta, E., Arango, C., DeTore, N. R., Eberlin, E. S., Mueser, K. T., & Correll, C. U. (2023, January). Efficacy and acceptability of psychosocial interventions in schizophrenia: Systematic overview and quality appraisal of the meta-analytic evidence. *Molecular Psychiatry, 28*(1), 354–368.

chapter 10

Managing treatment-related complications

Antipsychotic drugs (APDs), like all medicines, can cause side effects. For the majority of patients these are few and transient and should not prevent continued treatment. On the other hand, side effects require prompt attention to alleviate discomfort and prevent rare but more serious adverse reactions. Additionally, persistent side effects can contribute to treatment non-adherence (see Chapter 12), which increases the risk for decompensation and relapse. Therefore, one should be familiar with expected and common side effects, as well as serious and potentially permanent complications.

General principles

Observing the following principles (the '10 Cs' of optimal prescribing) can improve the chances of a favorable outcome and minimize treatment-related discomfort (Salzman et al., 2010).

- Collaboration: establish therapeutic alliance
- Comprehensive assessment, including medication and allergy history
- Consent for treatment, following psychoeducation
- Choose the right medicine for the given set of symptoms, co-morbid conditions and cost
- Complete the course of treatment (avoid switching APD prematurely)
- Compliance: check
- Comorbidities: evaluate

DOI: 10.4324/9781315152806-10

- Consider cost-effectiveness
- Consultations, as needed, for second opinion or medical reasons
- Chart notes: always provide treatment rationale in progress notes

JB is a young male admitted to the hospital for severe hallucinations and aggressive behavior. He was administered 5 mg haloperidol in the Emergency Room. He presents at the nursing station in obvious distress with his tongue sticking out and eyes rolling up.

JB is presenting with classic acute dystonia, with protruding tongue and oculogyric crisis (eyes locked upwards). Other presentations include spasms of the neck and trunk. Even laryngospasm can occur with breathing difficulties. Prompt treatment with intramuscular or intravenous benztropine 2 mg or diphenhydramine 50 mg; repeat after 10–15 minutes if no response. Usually there is prompt and dramatic relief. In those individuals at risk (young, male, high dose of typical APD), oral anticholinergic may be used prophylactically. Atypical APDs are a better choice in high-risk individuals.

What is going on?
What remedy will you offer?

The general side effects and range of severity for different antipsychotic medications are summarized Table 10.1, and approaches to management of common side effects are discussed in Table 10.2.

Table 10.1 General side effects of APDs and range of severity

	EPS TD	Dyslipidemia	Weight gain T2DM	Elevated prolactin	Anti-cholinergic Effects	Orthostatic hypotension	QTC prolongation
First generation*							
Chlorpromazine	+	+++	+++	++	+++	+++	+++
Haloperidol	+++	+	+	+++	+/-	-	++ (+++ If IV)
Fluphenazine	+++	+	+	+++	+/-	-	+/-
Second generation*							
Aripiprazole	+	-	+	-	-	-	+/-
Asenapine	++	-	++	++	-	+	++
Brexpiprazole	+	+	+	+/-	+/-	+/-	+/-
Clozapine	+/-	++++	++++	+/-	+++	+++	++
Lurasidone	++	+/-	+/-	+/-	-	+	+/-
Olanzapine	+	+++	+++	+	++	+	++
Paliperidone	+++	+	+++	+++	-	++	++
Quetiapine	+/-	+++	+++	+/-	++	++	++
Risperidone	+++	+	+++	+++	+	+	++
Ziprasidone	+	+/-	+/-	+	-	+	+++ (BBW!)

Table 10.2 Management of side effects (in alphabetical order)

Treatment-related problem	*What to do*
Agranulocytosis Granulocyte count falls below 500/mm³, leading to heightened risk of fatal infections	While most commonly associated with clozapine, it can occur with any APD. It is a life-threatening side effect. Agranulocytosis is a medical emergency that may require hospitalization, isolation, prophylactic antibiotics, granulocyte colony-stimulating factor and granulocyte-macrophage colony-stimulating factor
Akathisia Subjective feeling of motor restlessness (jitteriness) felt mostly in the legs, and discomfort. Usually seen early in treatment	Lower the dose of APD. Akathisia is not responsive to anticholinergic drugs; beta-blockers like propranolol are more effective. Benzodiazepines can also be helpful. Since akathisia is most commonly observed with first-generation APDs, switching to second-generation APDs, other than high doses of risperidone, may offer the best solution
Anorgasmia Inability to achieve orgasm. It is more prevalent in women	This is not reported frequently, despite being relatively common. Therefore, it is important to ask specifically about sexual side effects. Lowering the dose or changing the APD can be helpful. Sildenafil has been used successfully in antidepressant-induced anorgasmia
Blurred vision	The most common reason for blurred vision is the anticholinergic effect of some APDs. If these APDs cannot be avoided, then pilocarpine or bethanecol may be used
Constipation	A common problem due to anticholinergic effects, low fiber intake and sedentary lifestyle. It can be treated with increased fiber intake (bran, vegetables and fruits, psyllium), prunes, increased non-calorie fluid intake, stool softeners (docusate) and exercise. Laxatives should be used sparingly
Dry mouth (xerostomia; *xero,* **dry)**	It is due to anticholinergic effects of APDs. Switch to an alternative APD if possible. Otherwise, advise chewing sugar-free gum, sips of cold calorie-free fluids or ice chips. Pilocarpine rinse may be helpful

Dystonia
Acute painful contraction of muscles, usually affecting the tongue, neck, eyes and trunk and leading to protruding tongue, abnormal head position, grimacing, eyes rolling up and neck spasm

Initially treat with intramuscular or intravenous benztropine 2 mg or diphenhydramine 50 mg; repeat after 15 minutes if no response. Usually there is prompt and dramatic relief. Thereafter, continue oral anticholinergic treatment. Dystonia frequency has been reduced by decreasing use of first-generation APDs

Ejaculatory dysfunction
Inability or delayed ability to ejaculate, or retrograde ejaculation

Reduced dose of APD can be effective. Alternatively, switch to a second- or third-generation APD

Erectile dysfunction
Inability to achieve and maintain a penile erection

Lowering the dose or changing the APD can be helpful. Sildenafil and analogs have been used successfully in antidepressant-induced erectile dysfunction

Glucose metabolism abnormality
Abnormal glucose-tolerance test result, increased fasting glucose levels or frank diabetes mellitus

Impaired glucose tolerance, hyperglycemia and diabetes mellitus are observed primarily with second-generation APDs, particularly clozapine and olanzapine. Management includes switching APD, monitoring glucose levels, weight loss if indicated and hypoglycemic agents such as metformin

Hyperprolactinemia
Elevation of prolactin above 20 pg/l, caused by dopamine blockade. Chronic prolactin elevation can cause amenorrhea, galactorrhea, gynecomastia and possible loss of bone density

Common with first-generation antipsychotics as well as risperidone. Some APDs such as aripiprazole have a low propensity to induce hyperprolactinemia, so it is wiser to switch APDs rather than attempting treatment with dopamine agonists such as bromocriptine

Hyperthermia

Mild elevation of body temperature is common during initial treatment, particularly with clozapine, and can be treated with antipyretics. Persistent hyperthermia can be indicative of other serious conditions and should be promptly investigated

Table 10.2 Continued

Leukopenia Decrease in white blood cells, generally <4000 cells/mm³	It is usually transient but requires careful observation with repeated white blood counts because it may be a harbinger of agranulocytosis. If no other treatable causes can be found, a trial of lithium may be warranted
Libido decrease	Decreased libido can occur in 25–50% of patients. Switching APDs to a dopamine partial agonist such as aripiprazole can be helpful
Lipid abnormalities Desirable cholesterol level <200 mg/dl Triglyceride level <150 mg/dl	Elevations in triglyceride and cholesterol levels occur with second-generation APDs, particularly clozapine and olanzapine. The degree of elevation is not well correlated with weight gain. Switching to another APD, if feasible, along with conservative measures (weight loss, exercise, dietary changes) and lipid-lowering agents, can be helpful
Liver enzyme elevation Alanine transaminase range 15–45 U/l	Increases in liver enzymes, particularly transaminases, are common and transient. In the event of persistent elevations or clinical hepatotoxicity, prompt referral to gastroenterologist is required
Neuroleptic malignant syndrome NMS, is sudden onset of muscle rigidity and hyperthermia, along with altered consciousness, autonomic instability and elevations in white blood cells and creatine phosphokinase (CPK)	NMS is potentially fatal and can occur with practically all APDs. If NMS is suspected, assess promptly. If confirmed, immediately stop the APD and start supportive treatment (hydrate, lower body temperature, correct electrolyte imbalance). Dopamine agonists (e.g. bromocriptine) or dantrolene may be used. After recovery, a different APD (i.e. a second- or third-generation APD) can be re-introduced cautiously
Orthostatic hypotension Fall in blood pressure occurring while arising from a seated or lying position, accompanied by faintness and light-headedness	Generally transient, rarely lasting longer than four to six weeks. Commonsense measures include advice about standing up slowly, getting out of bed slowly, elevating the headrest and increasing fluid and salt intake. If conservative measures fail, fludrocortisone may be tried. *Epinephrine* is contraindicated
Parkinsonism Tremor, rigidity, brady-kinesia (slow movements) and shuffling gait	Most commonly seen with typical APDs. Dose reduction, along with anticholinergic agents (e.g. benztropine), is generally quite effective. Alternatively, switch to atypical APD

QTc prolongation

The QT interval, the duration of ventricular depolarization and repolarization, is normally 380–420 ms. QT prolongation >500 ms is associated with the development of cardiac dysrhythmias, particularly *torsades de pointes* that can lead to sudden death

Careful cardiac monitoring should be instituted with increased QTc interval, particularly in those individuals with a medical history suggestive of heart disease. It is best to switch APDs to those less likely to induce Q – Tc prolongation

Sedation

In most instances sedation is transient and lasts about two weeks. When it interferes with functioning, change the dosing to all at bedtime, reduce daytime dosing and, if unsuccessful, switch to a less-sedating APD. Modafinil may be helpful

Seizures

Usually occur with rapid escalation of APD dose, and in a dose-dependent manner with clozapine. In the case of clozapine, divided dosing may decrease the risk. Anticonvulsants may need to be used

Sialorrhea

Drooling or excessive salivation is the pooling of saliva beyond the margin of the lip. Common with clozapine, it is not transient

Patients find sialorrhea quite bothersome. It tends to worsen during sleep. A towel over the pillow can help with the physical discomfort. Anticholinergic agents (e.g. benztropine, atropine drops) are helpful

Tachycardia

Rapid heartbeat >100 beats/min

It is seen with APDs with higher anticholinergicity or due to orthostatic hypotension, and tends to be transient. If persistent, atenolol may be used

Tardive dyskinesia (TD)

Non-rhythmic choreiform (jerky) or athetoid (slow, writhing) movements typically affecting the tongue, lips, jaw, fingers, toes and trunk. TD can be transient or permanent

Stopping the APD and switching to an atypical APD (such as quetiapine, olanzapine or aripirazole) may provide some relief over the course of several months or longer. Transient worsening of TD can occur when the APD dose is reduced. Clozapine is effective in some cases of severe and persistent TD. Vesicular monoamine transporter (VMAT-2) inhibitors (valbenazone and deutetrabenazine) have been approved by FDA for TD

Table 10.2 Continued

Weight gain	APDs vary significantly in their effect on weight. Because atypical APDs are increasingly used as first-line treatment, weight gain with these drugs has garnered the most attention. Clozapine and olanzapine have the highest weight-gain potential, while ziprasidone has the least, although all antipsychotics have the potential to cause weight gain. It is prudent to initiate weight-management principles concurrently with treatment, which include education, nutritional counseling, exercise and lifestyle alterations. If these measures fail, then switch APD if clinically feasible. Controlling weight gain during treatment is a significant challenge, because it occurs within the context of a larger societal problem of increasing obesity. Other alternatives to consider include add-on medications like Metformin and a widening array of weight-loss drugs that are being tested for this indication (e.g. GLP-1 agonists like Liragultide and Semaglutide). Bariatric surgery can be a viable option and may require close collaboration with bariatric specialty clinics.
Body mass index (BMI) is weight in kilograms divided by square of height in meters Normal BMI: 18.5–24.9 Overweight: 25–29.9 Obese: >30	

Reference

Salzman, C., Glick, I., & Keshavan, M. S. (2010, December). The 7 sins of psychopharmacology. *Journal of Clinical Psychopharmacology, 30*(6), 653–655.

chapter 11

Suboptimal treatment response

When treatment fails to provide satisfactory resolution of the symptoms of schizophrenia, it is important to first ask whether *optimal* treatment is being provided. Optimal pharmacotherapy can be thought of as the appropriate and effective drug at an adequate dose for an adequate length of time with the least burden of side effects and treatment complexity.

One-third of patients with schizophrenia, unfortunately, do not respond satisfactorily to optimal treatment. It is important to note that satisfactory response does not mean the absence of *all* signs and symptoms of schizophrenia. In fact, treatment that achieves criteria for remission of mostly positive symptoms for several months (Andreasen et al., 2005) would be considered an excellent therapeutic response.

Researchers utilize a variety of criteria for treatment response, usually focused on the reduction of positive symptoms (hallucinations, delusions and thought disorder) as assessed by rating scales, such as the commonly used Brief Psychiatric Rating Scale (BPRS). International guidelines generally define treatment-resistant schizophrenia (TRS, an unfortunate term suggesting that it is the patient who is resisting treatment, which may not be the case) as a lack of response to at least two antipsychotic drugs in adequate dose and duration, when adherence criteria are met, and the diagnosis is not in question (Correll & Howes, 2021). As per the treatment response and resistance in psychosis (TRRP) guidelines, adequate dose is defined as at least a chlorpromazine equivalent of 600 mg per day, for an adequate duration of at least six weeks. Good adherence is defined as taking medications > 80% of the time as confirmed by at least two sources (e.g. collateral

DOI: 10.4324/9781315152806-11

history, medication blood levels). At a practical level, the estimation of therapeutic response in an individual patient is dependent on a combination of factors, such as reduction of most symptoms, acceptance of some residual symptoms and tolerability of treatment.

> BR is 38 years old and married, with long-standing schizophrenia. He is being treated with 20 mg of olanzapine. He has put on 5 kg (10 lb) in weight, but his laboratory tests do not indicate any metabolic side effects. The auditory hallucinations are infrequent. He remains uncomfortable in crowds but is able to commute to the job center where he works for a stipend.
>
> *Would you change his treatment – yes or no?*
>
> It is unlikely we would change BR's treatment at this time because he appears to be doing fairly well. However, we would consider changing treatment if the patient expresses concern about the weight gain, discomfort with crowds or cognitive deficits that prevent advancement in his job. If the concern is limited to the infrequent auditory hallucinations, we would carefully review the advantages of tolerating residual symptoms and the disadvantages of altering a fairly effective treatment regimen, urging that treatment not be changed at this time.

Response to treatment varies along a continuum, ranging from no response at all to a rapid, complete and sustained resolution of symptoms. Most patients have a treatment response that falls somewhere between the two extremes (Figure 11.1).

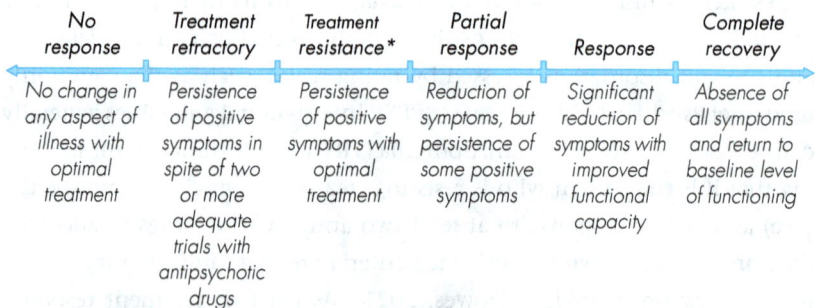

No response	Treatment refractory	Treatment resistance*	Partial response	Response	Complete recovery
No change in any aspect of illness with optimal treatment	Persistence of positive symptoms in spite of two or more adequate trials with antipsychotic drugs	Persistence of positive symptoms with optimal treatment	Reduction of symptoms, but persistence of some positive symptoms	Significant reduction of symptoms with improved functional capacity	Absence of all symptoms and return to baseline level of functioning

Figure 11.1 The treatment response continuum.

Causes of inadequate treatment response

CY is 33 years old, with recent-onset olfactory hallucinations, periods of fear and religious preoccupation. He has been treated with 4 mg of risperidone for two months. Although he has been adhering to his treatment, there has been no significant improvement in symptom severity.

What are your next steps?

In addition to reviewing the history of the illness, we would refer CY to a neurologist in order to rule out a neurological disorder. The recent-onset olfactory hallucinations, periods of fear and religious preoccupation are consistent with temporal-lobe disorders such as epilepsy. Risperidone may need to be continued to treat any residual psychosis. Antipsychotic drugs that lower the seizure threshold, such as clozapine, should be avoided.

When a suboptimal treatment response is encountered, the following questions are worth considering for each patient:

Right diagnosis? Right medication? In order for treatment to work, the prescribed medication needs to be appropriate for the condition in question. In other words, the treatment has to be appropriate for the patient's diagnosis. One caveat, however, should be borne in mind. Many medications, especially the atypical antipsychotic drugs, have beneficial effects across a variety of diagnostic categories, including the mood spectrum disorders. However, these medications are also widely prescribed in practice 'off label' to target symptoms (e.g. insomnia) or non-specific agitation in conditions for which there is weak or evidence of efficacy (e.g. autism spectrum disorders, anxiety, post-traumatic stress disorders). The clinician therefore has to first ask the question whether the diagnosis is right, while considering reasons for treatment resistance.

CR is a 26-year-old single mother with three young children who has been prescribed ziprasidone 40 mg BID, clozapine 50 mg BID, valproate 500 mg q AM and 250 mg at noon, 500 mg q HS and benztropine 1 mg BID. The severity of delusions of reference remains unchanged. Her memory is poor, and she often forgets if she took her medications.

What would you do?

CR has been prescribed a complicated regimen. The persistence of symptoms may indicate non-adherence with treatment. Missing or forgetting medications is an extremely common occurrence. The more complicated the medication regimen, the greater likelihood of missing a dose. The first task would be to simplify CR's medication regimen by following the **KISS** principle of pharmacotherapy (**K**eep **i**t **S**afe & **S**imple).

Was the medication taken by the patient? Even if the diagnosis and the prescribed treatment are correct, the patient may not be taking the medication as prescribed. The most common reason for this is treatment non-adherence. The factors that lead to non-adherence and approaches to address them are detailed in Chapter 12.

CR, the patient described above, has had her treatment regimen simplified. She is now taking clozapine 200 mg BID and valproate 500 mg BID. The delusions of reference are less bothersome, but she complains of constipation and is gaining weight.

What would you do?

CR appears to be responding to treatment, following the simplification of the treatment regimen and improved compliance. The inadequate sleep and weight loss may be new concerns or old concerns coming to light with the reduction in psychosis. Before considering any change in treatment, it is important to determine whether she's experiencing stress, a well-known cause of sleep and appetite disturbance. CR is a single mother with three young children. The absence of social supports or ill health in children can easily lead to increased stress, which can increase the risk of psychotic relapse.

Are psychosocial stressors compromising treatment response? In spite of seemingly optimal treatment there can be suboptimal response. After reassessing diagnosis and compliance, it is prudent to ask about stressors in a patient's life. It is well known that stress can increase the risk of decompensation and relapse. Likewise, stress can compromise ongoing treatment. Addressing specific psychosocial stressors (stress reduction) can be very helpful for the overall outcome and for improving specific treatment response.

Does the drug have optimum concentration in the body? Even when the medication prescribed is taken with good adherence, there are other reasons why adequate concentrations may not have been reached. Plasma concentrations depend on both the rate of dosing of a medication and its clearance by the body, generally by liver enzymes – cytochrome oxidases. The metabolic rate of a given drug may vary from person to person; some individuals metabolize at a faster rate (rapid metabolizers), others at a slower rate (slow metabolizers). At a given dose, rapid metabolizers will have lower plasma levels than slow metabolizers. Genetic factors, as well as physiological parameters (age, co-morbid illness, concurrent medications, diet and pregnancy), can affect the pharmacokinetics of medications, leading to alterations in plasma concentrations even when the dose is constant.

Examining plasma levels of some antipsychotics can inform dosing. The estimation of plasma levels of clozapine is most common (levels below 350 ng/ml are associated with reduced response and should thus support dose increase). Higher clozapine levels should suggest close monitoring for side effects such as seizures. Plasma norclozapine (an inactive metabolite of clozapine) levels are not correlated with treatment response but are useful in determining the metabolic rate of clozapine. The optimal ratio of clozapine/norclozapine for non-smokers is around 1.3. Lower ratios suggest more rapid metabolism, which can be induced by smoking.

Did the drug have the desired effect? Sometimes the desired effect of the drug is not occurring at specific receptors in the brain, in spite of adequate plasma concentrations. There are multiple reasons for lack of effect. Individual genetic differences in receptor affinities may exist, similar to genetic differences in drug metabolism. It turns out that many of the abovementioned factors affecting pharmacokinetics can also affect receptor responsivity to the drug. There is much ongoing research aimed at identifying these genetic variations in order to tailor treatments to the individual patient.

Approaches to suboptimal treatment response

'What do we do when nothing works?' is a common lament that all practicing clinicians will have to contend with when treating patients with schizophrenia. These are cases where interventions need to go beyond the current evidence base (i.e. guidance from scientific studies of populations). The

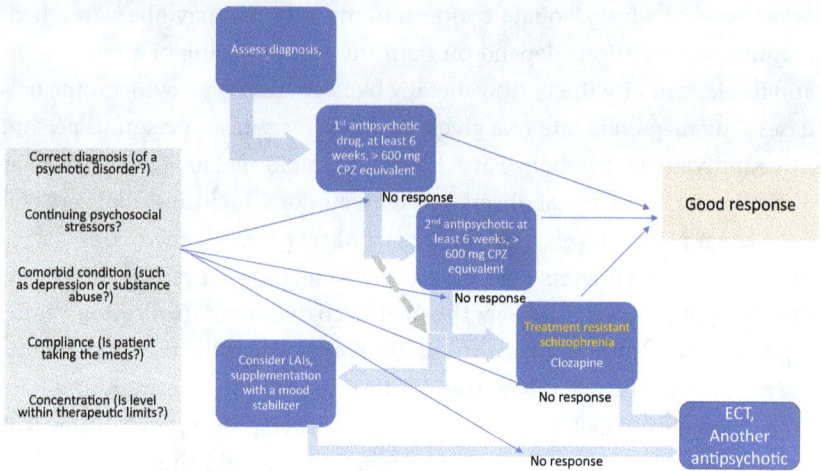

Figure 11.2 Optimizing treatment.

other sources of evidence are physiologic rationale and patient preferences and values that can together guide an empirical approach. Before embarking on empirical modification of treatment, it is worth reviewing once again for the presence of factors associated with suboptimal treatment response (wrong diagnosis, substance abuse, co-morbid disorders and psychosocial stressors). Next, serial trials of medications or combinations of medications can be attempted with careful follow-up and measurement of response and side effects (Figure 11.2). It is important to define clear targets and to discontinue and document unsuccessful trials (that either did not improve the target symptoms or caused unacceptable side effects), in order to avoid the unnecessary accumulation of medications that can increase the risk for interactions and cumulative side effects. Enrollment in clinical trials, when this option is available, may be the safest and most ethical option for a patient who would otherwise be subject to the uncontrolled and unscientific approach of serial trials in usual clinical practice.

Raise the dose

This was common practice in the 1970s and 1980s: the so-called high-dose and rapid neuroleptization strategies, which led to serious extrapyramidal complications while using typical antipsychotic drugs. The general thinking used to be that if you double the dose, you would have double the effect.

However, keep in mind that if a medication is ineffective for other reasons, raising the dose is unlikely to help and will increase the risk of side effects. The key concept to consider is achieving a minimum effective dose: that is, a dose that is effective but not high enough to cause side effects.

Lower the dose or try without it

Higher doses than recommended may diminish efficacy, because of side effects, and the wiser step may be to reduce the dose. For example, treating akathisia by lowering the antipsychotic dose can have salutary effects on psychosis severity. When there is lack of clarity, it may be worth considering a brief period off medication. Such medication-free trials carry significant risk of further worsening of the patient's condition and must be conducted in carefully controlled settings, such as the inpatient service.

Add another medication

It is a common practice to add either another antipsychotic or a mood stabilizer to an existing antipsychotic medication. While polypharmacy is generally not recommended, it may be useful to consider medication combinations, especially if the benefits are complementary and there are no additive side effects. For example, it is unwise to combine two medications that have similar side effects, such as weight gain (for example, olanzapine and quetiapine); on the other hand, combining a highly sedative antipsychotic such as clozapine with an activating antipsychotic such as aripiprazole may be worth considering in specific situations.

Switching to a new medication

If the current antipsychotic medication is convincingly ineffective, this is an appropriate approach. By and large it is better to consider interclass as opposed to intraclass switching of the medications. For example, it would make little sense to switch from trifluoperazine to perphenazine, both of which are phenothiazines. On the other hand, it may be worth considering a switch from a first-generation to a second- or third-generation antipsychotic drug.

Clozapine

If two or more antipsychotic medications have been found ineffective, the appropriate next step is to consider clozapine, if there are no contraindications.

Clozapine is the only antipsychotic approved by the Food and Drug Administration (FDA) for treatment-resistant schizophrenia (TRS). It is also approved for suicidality in schizophrenia or schizoaffective disorder, and is used off-label in bipolar disorder. Compared to first-generation antipsychotics, clozapine shows superior effects (small to medium effect sizes) on positive, negative and overall symptoms as well as relapse rates in TRS and treatment non-resistant schizophrenia. Hospitalization rates, mortality and all-cause discontinuation were also superior with clozapine. Clozapine is associated with several side effects, especially in the first several weeks. Most can be managed effectively without discontinuation. The most important to consider may be remembered as the ABCDEs:

- Agranulocytosis and Anticholinergic side effects
- Body weight increase
- Constipation and Cardiac side effects
- Drooling, Drowsiness and Diabetes risk and
- Epileptic Seizures

It is important to proactively assess, monitor and address side effects. In the US, plasma neutrophil counts must be monitored weekly during the first six months of treatment, followed by every other week for six months and monthly thereafter. Additional requirements through the clozapine risk evaluation and mitigation system (REMS) include prescriber and pharmacy certification, patient enrollment and routine submission of neutrophil counts. For a recent update on clozapine, the reader is referred to Keshavan et al. (2022).

Summary

- **Suboptimal treatment response** is when treatment fails to provide satisfactory resolution of the symptoms. One-third of patients with schizophrenia do not respond satisfactorily to optimal treatment.
- The assessment of therapeutic response in an individual patient is dependent on a combination of factors such as reduction of most symptoms, acceptance of some residual symptoms and tolerability of treatment.
- Response to treatment occurs along a continuum, ranging from no response at all to a rapid, complete and sustained resolution of symptoms.

- Questions to ask in the case of suboptimal treatment response are:
  - Right diagnosis? Right medication?
  - Was the medication taken by the patient?
  - Are psychosocial stressors compromising treatment response?
  - Does the drug have optimum concentration in the body?
  - Did the drug have the desired effect?
- **Causes of suboptimal treatment response** are not always apparent or even discoverable. Therefore, an empirical approach is required, informed by research evidence (summarized in Figure 11.1):
  - Raise the dose
  - Lower the dose or try without it
  - Add another medication
  - Switch to a new medication

References

Andreasen, N. C., Carpenter, W. T., Jr., Kane, J. M., Lasser, R. A., Marder, S. R., & Weinberger, D. R. (2005, March). Remission in schizophrenia: Proposed criteria and rationale for consensus. *American Journal of Psychiatry*, *162*(3), 441–449.

Correll, C. U., & Howes, O. D. (2021, September 7). Treatment-resistant schizophrenia: Definition, predictors, and therapy options. *Journal of Clinical Psychiatry*, *82*(5).

Keshavan, M. S., Bishop, D. L., Coconcea, C., & Bishop, J. R. (2022, October). Clozapine, an update. *Schizophrenia Research*, *248*, 168–170.

chapter 12

Medication nonadherence

Arguably one of the greatest challenges that a clinician will face in caring for the patient with schizophrenia is nonadherence to antipsychotic medication. It is paramount that the possibility of nonadherence be considered from initial treatment contact. Nonadherence is more common early in the course of schizophrenia. Lack of insight is the most common cause.

General principles

What is adherence?

Treatment adherence or compliance is taking medicine as prescribed, including at the dose, timing, frequency and duration specified. Treatment adherence also includes prescribed prohibitions, such as on driving or operating machinery or consuming alcohol, illicit drugs, specified foods or other substances. Any deviation from the prescribed regimen constitutes nonadherence.

How common is nonadherence?

Treatment nonadherence is relatively common across all medical specialties (Figure 12.1), but more so in persons with schizophrenia. (Nearly three-quarters of patients become non-adherent within two years following discharge.) Most clinicians underestimate treatment nonadherence.

DOI: 10.4324/9781315152806-12

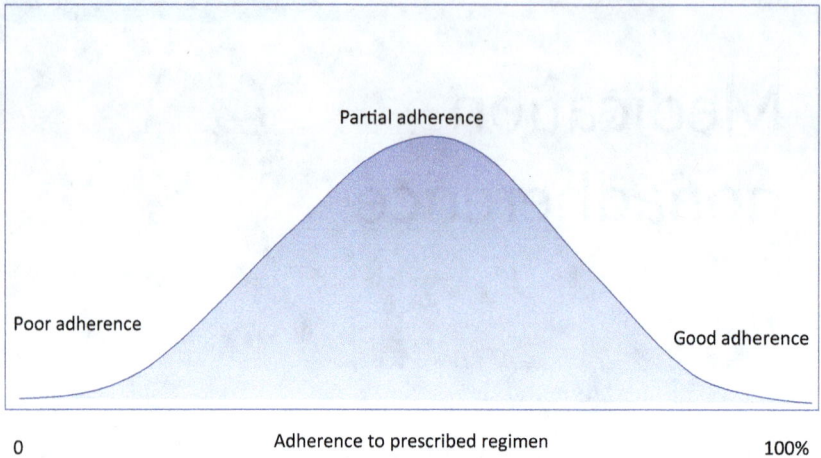

Figure 12.1 Degree of adherence varies widely among schizophrenia patients.

Why does nonadherence matter?

The consequences of nonadherence depend on its nature. Partial nonadherence can result in incomplete treatment response, increasing the risk of chronicity as well as relapse. There is also evidence that recurrent relapses can lead to more severe brain changes and functional declines in schizophrenia. With total nonadherence, relapse is very common, occurring in nearly 80% of patients within five years.

How do we assess nonadherence?

Since both clinicians and patients underestimate nonadherence, it is useful practice, particularly early in treatment, to rely on objective and practical methods, such as pill counts, for estimating treatment adherence. We recommend asking patients to bring their pill bottles with them to outpatient visits. It is also very useful to ask family members or support staff about adherence.

Suspect nonadherence when you note:
- unexplained change in behavior
- missed appointments

- evidence of substance abuse (smell of alcohol on breath, pupils that are dilated or pinpoint)
- the patient is beginning a new relationship – inquire especially about sexual side effects and the partner's views on medications and mental illness

What causes nonadherence?

There are many reasons why patients choose not to adhere to recommended treatment. Early in the course of illness, denial of illness is one of the commonest reasons. Medication side effects are another very common reason. Figure 12.2 outlines various causes of treatment nonadherence. Nonadherence is in most cases a decision made by the patient, after he/she weighs the perceived risks and benefits of treatment, as per the health belief model (Perkins, 1999). This model suggests that Health behaviors are best explained by the patients' perceived benefits vs disadvantages/barriers for health-related actions.

When faced with treatment nonadherence, each of the above factors must be considered. In fact, astute clinicians always keep these factors in mind when interacting with patients.

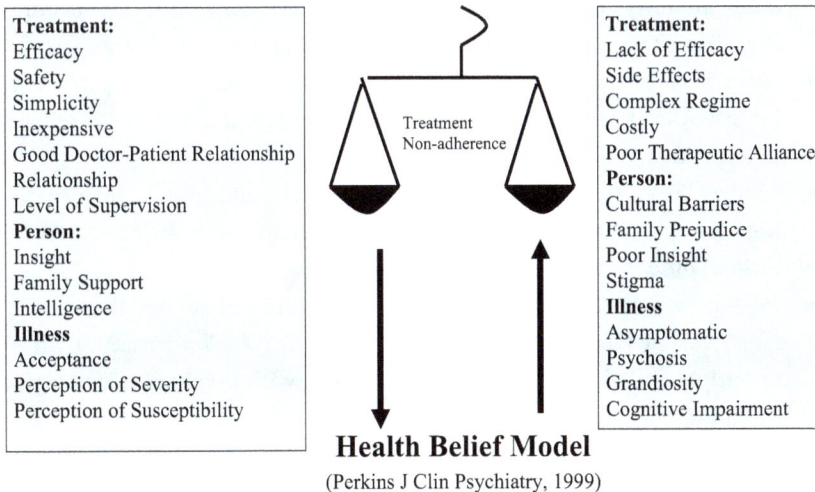

Treatment:
Efficacy
Safety
Simplicity
Inexpensive
Good Doctor-Patient Relationship
Relationship
Level of Supervision
Person:
Insight
Family Support
Intelligence
Illness
Acceptance
Perception of Severity
Perception of Susceptibility

Treatment Non-adherence

Treatment:
Lack of Efficacy
Side Effects
Complex Regime
Costly
Poor Therapeutic Alliance
Person:
Cultural Barriers
Family Prejudice
Poor Insight
Stigma
Illness
Asymptomatic
Psychosis
Grandiosity
Cognitive Impairment

Health Belief Model
(Perkins J Clin Psychiatry, 1999)

Figure 12.2 Causes of non-adherence in schizophrenia.

How do we manage nonadherence?

Management of treatment nonadherence depends on the factors that are operative in specific clinical situations, some of which are illustrated below. Strategies to address nonadherence can be *proactive* or *reactive* or both.

Proactive approaches presume that nonadherence occurs at very high rates and is nevertheless underestimated by both clinicians and patients. Being proactive should not interfere with the therapeutic alliance – it need not be viewed as mistrust of the patient's intentions.

Reactive approaches are instituted in the face of clear evidence of nonadherence.

An overarching set of principles in approaching treatment nonadherence has been articulated by Dr Xavier Amador (*I Am Not Sick: I Don't Need Help*, Vida Press, 2000). He calls it **LEAP** (**L**isten, **E**mpathize, **A**gree and **P**artner).

Additionally, common approaches to managing nonadherence include:

- *Lack of insight* is a prelude to nonadherence and withdrawal from treatment. Assess insight early and proactively institute plans to engage patient in treatment; invite assistance from family and friends
- *Improved treatment outcome*. Suboptimal therapeutic response is associated with high degrees of nonadherence. Patients can be unrealistic about rapidity of response or presence of residual symptoms. Realign their expectations to be consistent with general clinical experience
- *Side effects*. Proactively ask about side effects at each visit. Pay particular attention to sexual and cognitive side effects and treatment-related dysphoria
- *Simplify the treatment regimen*. Whenever possible, utilize bedtime or morning dosing, and preferably once daily. Ask patients about their preference
- *Reduce cost of medications* if this is an issue
- *Inquire about cultural, religious or social barriers* to treatment adherence
- *Inquire about family attitudes towards psychiatric medications*. Not infrequently, families discourage any association with psychiatry, leading to nonadherence by the patient
- *Feeling well*. Not surprisingly, patients who are recovered feel they no longer need treatment. This is the time to be vigilant: education regarding the risk of relapse without treatment must be reinforced

- *Grandiosity or florid psychosis.* When allying with the patient's delusions fails to engage them in treatment, then coercive treatments may be required if danger to the patient or others is unequivocally present

Common clinical scenarios

AC is a 31-year-old engineer who presents at the ER with a recent worsening of paranoia. He is prescribed 2 mg risperidone and discharged. He is not seen again at the outpatient clinic, but presents at the emergency room the following day believing he has 'meningitis'.

Why is the patient complaining about 'meningitis'? What management would you suggest?

AC was experiencing motor side effects (extrapyramidal side effects, particularly neck rigidity). Management includes lowering antipsychotic drug dose, treating the side effects with anticholinergic agents and switching antipsychotic, if possible, to one with a lower propensity for motor side effects.

Side effects are a very common reason for nonadherence. The clinician should be familiar with the usual side effects of medications they prescribe, and should communicate these to the patient with sensitivity and reassurance. Family members should also be informed of side effects so that they can help monitor the patient, particularly during the early days of treatment.

MK is a 28-year-old man discharged from the inpatient unit on Friday. On Monday, nurses noted that he forgot to take his follow-up instructions. He missed his appointment on Wednesday, but showed up a year later with a severe psychotic decompensation.

Why did he miss his appointment?

If you could go back in time, what would you do?

MK did not show up for his appointment likely because no therapeutic alliance was established prior to discharge and aggressive follow-up care was not instituted. To facilitate aftercare, therapeutic continuity should be enhanced, barriers to treatment should be assessed and letters should be written if phone contact is unsuccessful.

Patients miss appointments for many reasons, but a common one is lack of alliance with the clinician. It is vital that the patient be a partner in his or her care. This minimizes the possibility of nonadherence. Patients who appear not to care about their treatment should be closely monitored. While there are 'passive' patients who go along with treatment, they can just as easily slip out of treatment.

> BA is a 26-year-old woman with three young children who has been prescribed ziprasidone 40 mg BID, clozapine 50 mg BID, depakote 500 mg q AM and 750 mg q HS and benztropine 1 mg BID. One day, the police are called mid-day because she is not answering her door and the children are crying inside.
>
> *What do you think happened?*
>
> *How would you manage this medication regimen?*
>
> BA either decompensated, after not taking medication as prescribed, or accidentally overdosed. What BA needs is a simpler medication regimen (KISS – *Keep it Safe and Simple*).

Any barriers to taking medications should be identified and cues developed for taking medication. Tracking adherence, for example by checking refill dates or pill counting, can help the clinician intervene early.

Missing or forgetting medications is an extremely common occurrence in all of medicine, but particularly so in psychiatry. The more complicated the medication regimen, the greater the likelihood of missing a dose or overdosing. Imagine a scenario in which an otherwise diligent patient has to contend with three different medications over four different time-points daily. Simplify, simplify and simplify!

> JL, a 21-year-old college freshman, is admitted for 'odd' behavior after trying to climb the science building and patrolling the neighborhood at night in order to save lives. He does not believe he is ill and refuses all medications.
>
> *Why do you think JL is refusing medications? How would you get him to take medicines?*
>
> JL has no insight into the nature of his behavior or its consequences. First, actively listen to JL's concerns. This may help him feel understood and possibly improve the chances of JL listening to you in return! Elicit support from family and friends who may be able to influence his decisions. Obtain a second opinion if necessary. As a last resort, initiate the process for compulsory medication (if legally available) only if JL is a danger to himself or others.

Patients who refuse medications because they lack insight into the nature or severity of their illness are especially challenging to persuade to partner in their own care. Every effort should be made to get them to initiate treatment. Sometimes short-acting antianxiety agents can reduce the severity of the illness enough to permit negotiation regarding antipsychotic medications. Although there is a continuum of opinions regarding forced treatment, always bear in mind that any intervention must be in the patient's best interest.

> **STRONG FEELINGS!** Patients who refuse medications often generate strong feelings in treating staff. This stems from a sense of helplessness at not being able to compel a 'helpless' patient to comply with treatment, as well as feelings of anger at the patient for not 'cooperating'. While these feelings may appear understandable, they have the power to unconsciously distort relations with the patient in unhelpful ways. It is imperative that clinicians remind themselves that a patient who refuses treatment has an illness that underlies the behavior. Reframing a patient's 'obstinate' behavior in this way facilitates proactive and empathetic actions on his or her behalf.

> KC is a 34-year-old unemployed lawyer treated with olanzapine 40 mg daily for intractable beliefs that his family has been replaced by 'replicas'. During reevaluation, the clinician is puzzled about why KC has not put on any weight.
>
> *What are the key points to consider here?*
>
> *How would you facilitate treatment adherence?*
>
> It appears that the treatment offered has not been effective. Since olanzapine is associated with some weight gain, its absence raises the possibility of nonadherence. Assess compliance: if KC has been compliant with treatment, then titrate the olanzapine dose and ensure an adequate duration of treatment; if still no response, attempt augmentation strategies or change the antipsychotic prescribed.

Long-acting depot antipsychotic agents (LAIs)

Compared to oral antipsychotics, the advantages of LAIs include improved adherence, reduced relapse and hospitalization risk and the ability to differentiate true treatment resistance from 'pseudo'-resistance (Haddad & Correll, 1999). Additionally, LAIs are associated with lower all-cause mortality than OAs. LAIs are under-utilized in most clinical settings in the US; reasons may include negative attitudes, misconceptions and lack of knowledge among clinicians, patients and carers. Practical barriers to LAI use include acquisition costs and inadequate service structures to administer/monitor LAI treatment.

Patients often view the suggestion for using depot antipsychotics quite negatively, because it may indicate to them that:

- they cannot be trusted to comply with oral medications
- the patient is a 'tough' case and requires more 'serious' treatment
- the doctor (and often society, by extension) is taking away his or her liberty to refuse treatment or choose the kind of treatment
- the doctor wants to punish the patient

However, depot antipsychotics do offer a variety of advantages:

- patients receive prescribed doses
- predictable and stable plasma concentrations
- efficacy with lower doses
- no risk of abrupt discontinuation
- rapid identification of nonadherence
- greater privacy in medication administration
- bypass effects of rapid metabolism

Recent evidence suggests that LAIs are effective for treating first-episode psychosis and for early initiation of treatment for schizophrenia (Figure 12.1). LAIs should not be restricted to patients with adherence problems, but instead should be more widely prescribed. LAIs should systematically be offered to all patients through shared decision-making. Any patient for whom long-term treatment is indicated should be considered a candidate for an LAI. Even if patients initially refuse an LAI, it is helpful to discuss it further to better understand the potential advantages. A common reason for non-acceptance of LAI therapy may be that psychiatrists are ambivalent or unenthusiastic about this option even as they recommend it.

An important barrier to success in addressing nonadherence is clinicians' tendency to emphasize obedience to medication rather than shared goals for decision-making toward optimal outcomes. Schizophrenia patients are

Table 12.1 Choosing an LAI antipsychotic: key considerations

Concern →	Cardio-metabolic	Prolactin	Less need for oral overlap	Fewer injections	Cost
Long-acting injectable **Consider**					
Aripiprazole	✓	✓			
Fluphenazine	✓✓				
Haloperidol	✓✓	✓			
Olanzapine			✓	✓	
Paliperidone			✓✓	✓✓	✓
Risperidone				✓	✓

Table 12.2 Strategies for managing treatment nonadherence

The problem	What to do
Patient refuses medications	Improve therapeutic alliance; rapid acting medications; involuntary medications as last resort
Patient is non-adherent because medications are not working	Dosage adjustment; consider medication switch, clozapine
Patient is non-adherent because of side effects	Dosage adjustment; consider medication switch; monitor & educate regarding side effects
Patient does not show up for first appointment	Improve hospital-to-clinic continuity; make care more accessible and patient-friendly
Patient who frequently misses/forgets medications or appointments	Cues to remember; memory aids such as pillboxes and alarm watches; phone call reminders; depot medication
Patient believes he/she does not need medications	Compliance therapy; continuing psychoeducation; cognitive remediation

often reluctant to disclose nonadherence because of the social risks involved in the therapeutic relationship. Nondisclosure leads the clinician to have insufficient information, leading to errors in treatment decisions. Adherence struggles could potentially interfere with the therapeutic relationship. It is important to address potential nonadherence at the beginning of treatment and provide the patient a 'safe corridor' to disclose likely medication lapses. It is important to focus on harm-reduction strategies to mitigate risks while seeking to to preserve the therapeutic relationship (Weiden, 2016).

Summary

- Nonadherence, ranging from partial to total, is common in schizophrenia.
- There are multiple causes of nonadherence, which may be related to the patient, the treatment or the illness; in most cases, the patient chooses not to adhere to treatment.

- Treatment of nonadherence needs to be guided by an understanding of the underlying causes of nonadherence.
- Long-acting injectable antipsychotic medications are effective in addressing nonadherence, and can improve outcomes even in patients without nonadherence.

References

Haddad, P. M., & Correll, C. U. (1999). Long-acting antipsychotics in the treatment of schizophrenia: Opportunities and challenges. *Expert Opinion on Pharmacotherapy, 24*(4), 473–493.

Perkins, D. O. (1999). Adherence to antipsychotic medications. *Review Journal of Clinical Psychiatry, 60*(Suppl. 21), 25–30.

Weiden, P. J. (2016, June). Redefining medication adherence in the treatment of schizophrenia: How current approaches to adherence lead to misinformation and threaten therapeutic relationships. *Psychiatric Clinics of North America, 39*(2), 199–216.

chapter 13

Managing decompensation and relapse

Schizophrenia tends to have a lifelong course. This does *not* mean that individuals with schizophrenia cannot have good recovery with a high quality of life. However, for many patients the course of illness is beset with episodes of decompensation and relapse. The challenge for the patient and clinician is to minimize the frequency and severity of relapse. It is well known that each episode of relapse becomes harder to treat than the previous one.

Decompensation We define decompensation as clinical worsening from current level of stability that does not meet criteria for relapse; it is transitory and fluid. The patient can spontaneously return to a previous level of stability without active intervention or progress to a relapsed state. We find it useful to distinguish decompensation from relapse; this allows us to track clinical changes that merit careful monitoring.

Relapse While there are a variety of research criteria for relapse (e.g. 25% worsening from baseline), in general it is understood as clinical worsening that requires active intervention, ranging from adjustment of antipsychotic drug (APD) dose to increased level of care, such as more frequent emergency room visits or partial or inpatient hospitalization. About one-fifth of patients develop Breakthrough Psychosis even while on Antipsychotic Maintenance Medication.

Prediction of relapse

Early in the course of illness it can be difficult to predict the likelihood of relapse. Just as the clinician is likely to be on firmer ground when attempting to predict a second episode in someone who has already had a first

DOI: 10.4324/9781315152806-13

episode, subsequent episodes become easier to predict as patterns emerge in the context of repeated relapse. However, there are a number of factors, some patient-related and others environmental, that typically conspire to worsen the clinical state. Some factors, such as life events, can be transient, which may lead to decompensation and possibly spontaneous return to baseline with the passing of the disturbing life event (Emsley et al., 2013). Relapse can be precipitated by a single factor but is often the result of the snowballing effect of multiple risk factors, which are shown in Figure 13.1.

Factors associated with RELAPSE are:

- **Relapse history** predicts subsequent relapses
- **Expressed emotion** (criticism or over-involvement), particularly by family members, predisposes to relapse
- **Life events**, both positive and negative, commonly precede relapse. Breakdown in relationships, eviction from home, loss of a job, poor grades in school are some examples
- **Alcohol and substance abuse (especially cannabis)** is a very common reason for relapse
- **Physical illnesses** that are concomitant, such as infections, new head injury, seizures or nutritional impairment can lead to worsening of symptoms

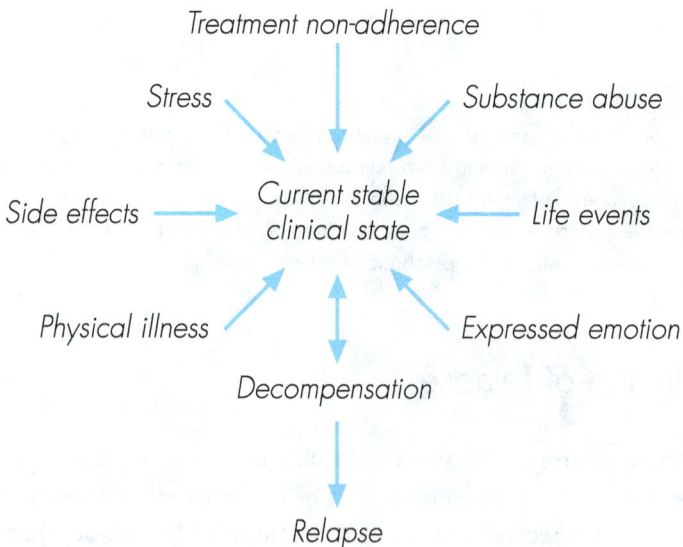

Figure 13.1 Decompensation and relapse risk factors.

- **Stopping medications** is by far the most common reason for relapse
- **Emergent side effects** such as akathisia, which used to be a quite common reason for relapse, fortunately decreased with the advent of atypical antipsychotic drugs (APDs)

Several of these factors are reversible or preventable. Discussing these predictors of relapse candidly with a patient, particularly during the first episode of psychosis, can go a long way in preventing relapse. As a simple tool for remembering the key reasons for relapse, patients and their families should be informed of the four S's: Early warning **Signs and Symptoms, Stress, Substance abuse** and **Stopping medications**.

It is important to develop, with the assistance of the patient and family, a list of **early warning symptoms** that are harbingers of relapse (Table 13.1). Each patient will have unique paths to decompensation or relapse. For one patient, the early warning sign may be the emergence of sleep difficulty, while in another patient it may be the return of auditory hallucinations. Smartphone applications such as MindLamp can help track early warning symptoms and predict relapse (Henson et al., 2021).

Management of decompensation

The challenge in managing decompensation is deciding when to take a stance of watchful inaction versus active intervention, because mild worsening of clinical state may simply be normal variation in response to life's vicissitudes, and the patient may return to the previous state relatively quickly. Acting too quickly and aggressively can be demoralizing to the patient; it engenders a feeling that they are completely at the mercy of the healthcare system with no capability to manage the illness on their own. On the other hand, when the rate of decompensation is rapid, it is best to act quickly.

In patients having multiple relapses, the 'march' of clinical worsening towards relapse tends to be similar from one episode to the next. Thus, knowing well the psychiatric history of the patient is critical in deciding when and how to respond to change in clinical state. Also, a good therapeutic relationship with the patient and family is critical to successful relapse-prevention interventions.

Table 13.1 Early warning signs of impending relapse

Behavior	Feelings	Thoughts	Perception and cognition
Sleep difficulty	Helpless or useless	Thoughts are racing	Senses seem sharper
Speech jumbled/odd use of words	afraid of losing one's mind	Thinking one has special powers	Experiencing strange sensations
Talking or smiling to oneself	sad or low	Thinking one can read other's minds	Hearing voices
Acting suspiciously as if being watched	anxious and restless	Thinking other people can read one's mind	Seeing visions or things others cannot see
Odd behavior	increasingly religious	Receiving personal messages from TV/radio	Thinking that a part of body has changed shape
Isolative	like being watched	Difficulty making decisions	Difficulty concentrating
Neglecting one's appearance	Fatigued	Preoccupied	Difficulty remembering things
Acting like one is somebody else	Confused	Thinking he/she might be somebody else	
Not eating	Forgetful	Thinking people are talking about him/her	
Not leaving the house	Unusually strong and powerful	Thinking people are against him/her	
Drinking more	Unable to cope	Bizarre thoughts	
Smoking more	like being punished	Thinking one's thoughts are controlled	
Movements are slow	Can't trust others		
Unable to sit still	Irritable		
Aggressive behavior	like you do not need sleep		
	Remorseful		

Adapted from: Birchwood M, Smith J, Macmillan F, et al. (1989)

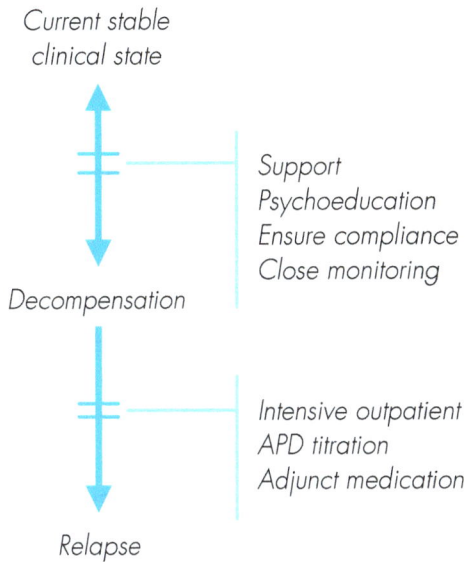

Figure 13.2 Interventions aimed at reversing decompensation and preventing relapse.

Measures that can reverse decompensation (Figure 13.2) include:

- supportive therapy to reinforce established coping approaches
- case management to assist with living situations that may be stressful
- psychoeducation to reinforce the goals of treatment
- ensuring treatment adherence, because clinical worsening can be both a consequence and a cause of treatment non-adherence

If decompensation is clearly heading towards a relapse, then initiate:

- intensive outpatient program (partial hospitalization)
- medication titration
- adjunctive medication (e.g. benzodiazepines)
- hospitalization, if required

Management of relapse

The management of relapse is the management of an acute episode. The steps taken to prevent a full-blown relapse may be helpful in mitigating the severity and duration of the relapse. Because each episode of relapse is more difficult to treat than the previous episode, it is worthwhile to spend considerable effort in preventing relapses. With each relapse comes the responsibility of devising an even better program of relapse prevention for the patient.

Relapse prevention

After the first episode of psychosis, the task of treatment is to keep the patient well for as long as possible. Thus, preventing relapses is the goal of maintenance treatment. Everything we have discussed about treatment so far is applicable to relapse prevention. However, framing these treatments as a formal program (and giving it a name) helps keep the focus on active prevention of relapse, not just treatment as usual.

Educating the patient and family about early signs and symptoms associated with relapse goes a long way towards relapse prevention. As noted above, each patient will have a unique pattern of relapse that tends to be the same for each episode. Table 13.1 contains a very comprehensive listing of early warning signs, developed by Birchwood and colleagues (1989).

Summary

- The course of schizophrenia illness for many patients involves episodes of decompensation (transitory clinical worsening) and relapse (clinical worsening that requires active intervention). The goal of maintenance treatment is to minimize the frequency and severity of relapse.
- Each episode of relapse becomes harder to treat than the previous one.
- A variety of factors are predictive of relapse and increase its risk: **relapse history, expressed emotion, life events, alcohol and substance abuse, physical illnesses, stopping medications** and **emergent side effects.** Discuss these predictors with patients and families at the beginning of treatment.
- Identify early warning symptoms that are unique to given patient.
- Management of decompensation involves taking a stance of watchful inaction in the case of mild worsening of clinical state. Act quickly when the rate of decompensation is rapid. Knowing well a patient's psychiatric history can help in deciding when and how to respond to change in

clinical state. Give appropriate supportive therapy, apply case management and psychoeducation and encourage treatment adherence.

- A good therapeutic relationship with the patient and family is critical to successful relapse-prevention interventions.
- Relapse prevention can involve an intensive outpatient program, medication titration, adjunctive medication or hospitalization.
- Relapse management is similar to the management of an acute episode.

References

Birchwood, M., Smith, J., Macmillan, F., Hogg, B., Prasad, R., Harvey, C., & Bering, S. (1989). Predicting relapse in schizophrenia: The development and implementation of an early signs monitoring system using patients and families as observers, a preliminary investigation. *Psychological Medicine, 19*, 649–656.

Emsley, R., Chiliza, B., Asmal, L., & Harvey, B. H. (2013). The nature of relapse in schizophrenia. *BMC Psychiatry, 13*, 50.

Henson, P., D'Mello, R., Vaidyam, A., Keshavan, M., & Torous, J. (2021, January 11). Anomaly detection to predict relapse risk in schizophrenia. *Translational Psychiatry, 11*(1), 28.

chapter 14

Suicide and violence

Suicide

Schizophrenia is a disorder with quite high mortality. About half of all patients with schizophrenia attempt suicide and 2–5% of patients die from suicide (Hor & Taylor, 2010; Dutta et al., 2010). Despite advances in treatment over the last half-century, the rates of suicide and parasuicide (suicide attempts) have not declined. Thus, suicide assessment and prevention are an important component in the treatment of schizophrenia.

Risk factors

A variety of risk factors are associated with suicide in general and schizophrenia in particular, and the two sets do not necessarily overlap. For example, being male is a risk factor for suicide in the general population but a less robust predictor of suicide in the case of schizophrenia. Predictors of suicide in schizophrenia include high premorbid IQ and good premorbid achievement predisposing to failed expectations and early relapse or disability leading to a fear of mental deterioration; psychological factors include hopelessness, perceived loss of control over the illness and experience of stigma. The risk of a suicide attempt during the first year of treatment is as high as 10%. The following are established risk factors for schizophrenia (SADHEART):

DOI: 10.4324/9781315152806-14

Single
Alcohol and substance abuse
Depressed mood
Hopelessness
Early phase of illness
Achievement (high premorbid)
Recurrent relapses
Treatment nonadherence and treatment resistance

Also, suicide risk in schizophrenia is greatest 'early':

- Earlier (i.e., younger) age
- Early age at onset of illness
- Early phase of illness
- Early after recovery from first episode of illness
- Early after inpatient discharge; risk of completed suicide is greatest during the immediate post-discharge period
- Early low-level suicide ideation may predict later suicidality

The clinician should be vigilant for subtle and early indications of suicidality, monitor such patients closely, and institute appropriate interventions. Easy-to-use scales such as the patient health questionnaires (PHQ-9, item 9) can be used to identify suicide risk and can help initiate a conversation with patients to explore suicidal ideation and behavior further in the clinical setting. The three-digit 988 Suicide and Crisis Lifeline (supported by local and state sources as well as the Substance Abuse and Mental Health Services Administration [SAMHSA]) is now available as a national network of more than 200 crisis centers with confidential 24/7 support to people in suicidal crisis or mental-health-related distress (www.samhsa.gov/find-help/988). The patient and family should be made aware of these resources as part of a risk-mitigation strategy that empowers them to seek help when risk is elevated and also communicates the clinician's inability to reliably predict future risk.

This inability to predict risk should be straightforwardly communicated to families and patients in order to invite their collaboration in an ongoing effort to mitigate risk (Cole-King, 2013), by paying regular attention to emerging risk and addressing ongoing risk in an open and iterative manner that includes all members of a patient's community. Clinicians should be seen as one, but certainly not the only, resource available to assist the patient at times of crisis where interventions to delay self-harm (e.g., by brief admission to an emergency setting) may be all that is required to establish safety and revise a treatment plan.

Psychosocial interventions play an important role in the management of suicide risk, especially interventions to help coping with stress, loneliness and interpersonal/family conflicts. Clozapine in recent years has emerged as an important tool in the therapeutic armamentarium for suicidal behavior.

Violence

Given the portrayals in the media, one would naturally conclude that patients with schizophrenia routinely indulge in violent behavior. Although this is not the case, the data suggests there is an increased risk (Whiting et al., 2022). Aggression is best conceptualized as an accompaniment to irritability, loss of impulse control and neurological dysfunction, which is seen with many neurological and psychiatric disorders. However, the enduring image that patients with schizophrenia are prone to unpredictable violence has done a great disservice to them. When some patients exhibit aggressive behavior, it is often a result of bizarre hallucinations or delusions.

It is useful to view violence as either transient or persistent, because such a classification has management implications.

Transient violence occurs in the context of excitation and hyperarousal, usually in the midst of an acute episode of psychosis, particularly when leading up to or during hospitalization. Once the episode of psychosis is treated, the violence recedes and there is generally no continued aggressive behavior as long as treatment is continued and effective.

Persistent violence is committed by a very small proportion of patients with schizophrenia. Unlike transiently violent patients, these patients remain at high risk for violent behavior, even when receiving adequate treatment and not in a state of hyperarousal.

Risk factors for violent behavior (predicting DANGER) are

Delusions
Antisocial traits
Neurologic impairment

Gender – male
Ethanol and drug use
Repeated violence

However, these risk factors, even in combination, are poorly predictive of actual risk in a specific patient. Often there are idiosyncratic risk factors unique to a particular patient (Crighton, 2011). Thus, there is no substitute for a deep knowledge of and alliance with your patient.

Management of violence

Violence is a medical emergency. The first order of business is physical safety of all the parties. Verbal de-escalation and environmental modification are the first choice of intervention, and physical restraint is to be used only as last resort. For a detailed approach to managing agitation in psychotic disorders see Vieta et al. (2017). A quick but careful assessment should be performed to determine contributors to violence, particularly medical conditions. With a working diagnosis in hand, appropriate interventions can be instituted, which may include parenteral benzodiazepines (such as lorazepam) or antipsychotic drugs (APDs) such as haloperidol. Short-acting forms of other antipsychotics are also available, such as ziprasidone IM, asenapine sublingual and risperidone M tabs.

Once the violence has abated and treatment is underway, the episode(s) of violence should be reviewed in order to determine whether it was transient or possibly persistent. If transient, then no specific violence management may be required other than ensuring continued treatment. On the other hand, if the violence appears to be enduring, review of current pharmacological treatment and enrollment into a violence-prevention program is necessary. Atypical APDs, particularly clozapine, have been found to reduce violent behavior. Violence-reduction programs vary considerably, but most have the following components:

- cueing (identify signs of anger)
- cognitive behavior therapy
- cognitive remediation
- anger management
- coping skills
- relaxation techniques

- structured environment
- leisure activities

Summary

- Half of all patients with schizophrenia attempt suicide and 2–5% of patients die from suicide.
- A variety of risk factors are associated with suicide in schizophrenia: single status, alcohol and substance abuse, depressed mood, hopelessness, early phase of illness, high premorbid achievement, revolving-door admissions and treatment failure.
- Suicide risk in schizophrenia is greatest early in the course of illness, at a younger age and during the post-discharge period, and it is associated with low-level suicidal ideation.
- With regard to violence, patients with schizophrenia are at risk for periods of transient aggression (often related to untreated or poorly treated illness or comorbid substance use), that likely accounts for the small increased population-level risk for violence.
- Aggression is an accompaniment of irritability, loss of impulse control and neurological dysfunction.
- Violence can be **transient** or **persistent.** Transient violence is seen with excitation and hyperarousal, and with treatment it is controlled. Persistent violence is committed by a very small proportion of patients with schizophrenia; it can occur even when receiving adequate treatment and not in hyperarousal state.
- A variety of risk factors are predictive of violence. One of the most robust predictors is the previous history of violence. Others include persecutory delusions, lack of insight, substance abuse and treatment non-adherence; neurologic impairment and antisocial traits are associated with persistent violence, and male gender predisposes. There is no substitute to knowing and intervening on risk factors in or outside this list for your patient. We are better at preventing violence (towards oneself or others) with clinical interventions than we are at predicting the same violence.
- Violence is a medical emergency and management includes seeing to the physical safety of all the parties, quick but careful assessment and pharmacological interventions (benzodiazepines, droperidol or haloperidol).

References

Cole-King, A. (2013). Suicide mitigation: A compassionate approach to suicide prevention. *Advances in Psychiatric Treatment, 19*(4), 276–283.

Crighton, D. (2011, August). Risk assessment: Predicting violence. *Evidence-Based Mental Health, 14*(3), 59–61.

Dutta, R., Murray, R. M., Hotopf, M., Allardyce, J., Jones, P. B., & Boydell, J. (2010, December). Reassessing the long-term risk of suicide after a first episode of psychosis. *Archives of General Psychiatry, 67*(12), 1230–1237.

Hor, K., & Taylor, M. (2010, November). Suicide and schizophrenia: A systematic review of rates and risk factors. *Journal of Psychopharmacology, 24*(Suppl. 4), 81–90.

Vieta, E., Garriga, M., Cardete, L., Bernardo, M., Lombraña, M., Blanch, J., Catalán, R., Vázquez, M., Soler, V., Ortuño, N., & Martínez-Arán, A. (2017). Protocol for the management of psychiatric patients with psychomotor agitation. *BMC Psychiatry, 17*, 328.

Whiting, D., Gulati, G., Geddes, J. R., & Fazel, S. (2022, February 1). Association of schizophrenia spectrum disorders and violence perpetration in adults and adolescents from 15 countries: A systematic review and meta-analysis. *JAMA Psychiatry, 79*(2), 120–132.

chapter 15

Achieving recovery

All the information in the preceding chapters lays the foundation for helping patients achieve recovery. The **Recovery** concept has evolved in response to the experiences of people with mental illness. It involves a shift away from traditional clinical definitions, such as avoiding relapse, towards new priorities of supporting the person in working towards their own goals and taking responsibility for their own life. There are three types of recovery (Figure 15.1).

Syndromal recovery occurs when the patient is no longer in the pre-defined syndromal episode such as psychosis. **Functional recovery** implies that the patient will return to his or her most functional period prior to the onset of the disorder. This type of recovery is often slower and may require different interventions such as psychosocial and cognitive rehabilitation. **Personal recovery** refers to the unique process of changing one's attitudes, values, feelings, goals, skills and/or roles toward living a satisfying, hopeful and contributing life, despite the limitations caused by serious mental illness. This aspect of recovery can be summarized in the CHIME framework for personal recovery (Connectedness, Hope, Identity, Meaning and Empowerment) (Slade et al., 2014).

Having very modest aims for recovery (e.g. absence of positive symptoms as the only criterion) can be limiting, because all options for helping the patient may not have been considered. On the other hand, excessively rapid or lofty expectations that are not achieved can lead to demoralization. The most sensible approach is an individualized one. For each patient

DOI: 10.4324/9781315152806-15

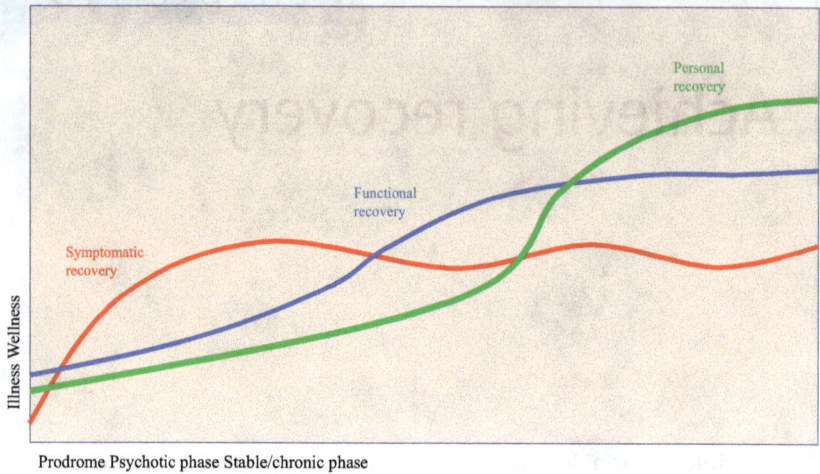

Prodrome Psychotic phase Stable/chronic phase

Figure 15.1 Three aspects of recovery in serious mental illness.

there are unique, interacting factors (similar to the 'epidemiological triad' of agent, host and environment) that influence the extent of recovery (Figure 15.2). These may be categorized as **disease-related** (e.g. illness severity, age of onset) **host-related** (e.g. patient's genetic liability), **environmental** (e.g. family interaction, substance exposure) and **treatment-related** (e.g. appropriate antipsychotic drug [APD] dose).

Recent research indicates that the following ten factors are important for achieving recovery:

Access to care. Continuous treatment and multimodal approaches (APDs, individual and group therapy, rehabilitation) are critical to achieving recovery.

Cognitive abilities. Adequate cognitive skills (working memory, perception skills and problem-solving abilities) are predictive of recovery.

Duration of untreated psychosis. Delay in treatment of the initial episode is associated with greater difficulty in achieving remission and can negatively impact long-term outcome.

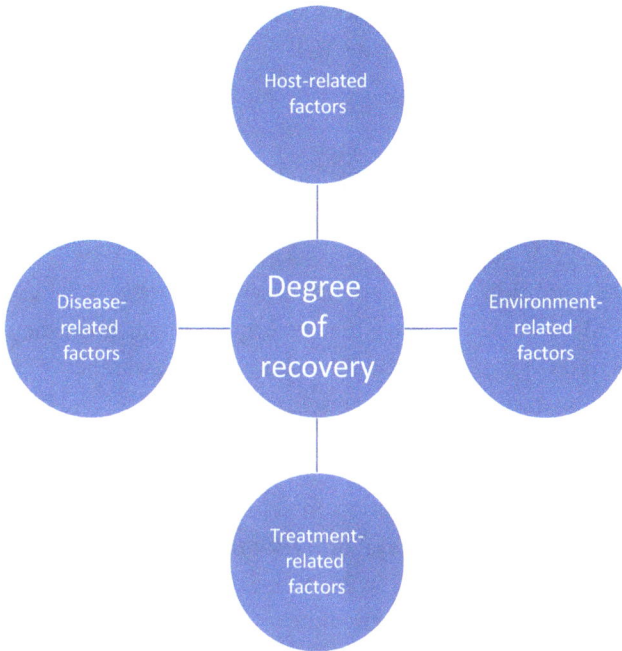

Figure 15.2 Relations between factors influencing recovery.

Family relationships. Family emotional support decreases relapse rate, while family stress increases the risk for relapse.

Initial response to medication. The rapidity of treatment response is a predictor of good outcome. Most patients with successful outcome report good response to the first APD used.

Personal history. Later age at onset of illness and good premorbid functioning are associated with recovery. Patients who have good outcome tend to have a higher IQ, a college degree and good work history.

Substance abuse. Almost half of the patients abuse substances (see below), which is associated with relapse and poorer outcome.

Social skills. Serious deficits in social skills are associated with unfavorable outcome.

Supportive therapy. Almost all patients who recover report being in regular therapy and having positive relations with clinical team members.

Treatment adherence. As has been mentioned throughout the book, non-adherence does not bode well for short-term remission and long-term recovery.

Co-morbid conditions

A variety of conditions are commonly observed together (co-morbid) with schizophrenia that significantly impact on treatment, outcome and, ultimately, recovery. Thus, there should be heightened awareness of these conditions when assessing and treating schizophrenia.

Depression

Depressive symptoms are common in schizophrenia and may be part of the prodrome or the florid phase, or follow the first episode (postpsychotic depression). Depression occurs in 25–40% of patients and is associated with increased suicidality and poor outcome.

The relationship between depression and schizophrenia has not been fully elucidated. Depression in schizophrenia may be due to the appearance of insight about the nature of illness and its lifetime implications. It may be integral to the schizophrenia illness or reflect another disorder such as schizoaffective disorder or major depression co-occurring with schizophrenia. First-episode patients tend to have more severe depression compared with multi-episode patients. Persistent hopelessness at discharge is associated with poorer outcome a year later.

Depressive symptoms seen in patients with schizophrenia present a diagnostic challenge. Depression accompanying psychosis is seen in major depression and the depressive phase of bipolar disorder. Neuroleptic-induced parkinsonism and primary negative symptoms can be mistaken for depression.

Co-morbid depression must be treated promptly. Selective serotonin reuptake inhibitors (SSRIs) are quite effective in treating depression in schizophrenia, unlike the older antidepressants. In the case of antidepressant-resistant depression, atypical APDs, particularly clozapine, have been helpful – more so than typical APDs.

Substance abuse

Substance abuse is very common in patients with schizophrenia; as many as half of all patients will abuse substances during their lifetime. The most common are nicotine and alcohol, followed by cannabis and cocaine. Cannabis misuse has increased significantly in recent years in the US; our studies suggest that over three-fourths of young, early-course patients use cannabis. Earlier age at first exposure to cannabis is associated with younger age at prodrome and psychosis onset and worse premorbid functioning (Kline et al., 2022). Dual diagnosis (substance abuse + schizophrenia) is more common in young males with lower education. Family history of substance abuse and conduct disorders further increase the risk for substance abuse.

Substance abuse can precede, accompany or follow the first psychotic episode. The physiological effects of abused substances tend to occur at much lower quantities in patients with schizophrenia. The course of substance abuse in schizophrenia tends to be chronic, with multiple relapses. Substance abuse has many dire consequences, including:

- higher relapse rates
- treatment non-adherence
- blunting of APD effectiveness
- violence
- depression
- suicide
- increased risk of injury and medical illness
- financial problems
- legal problems
- housing problems
- increased use of emergency services

Achieving abstinence is not easy and requires an integrated approach to assessment and treatment. The most important component of assessment is screening for substance abuse. This includes asking patients directly about substance abuse, urine drug screening and collateral sources of information. Treatment consists of psychoeducation, enhancing motivation to quit (motivational interviewing), psychological interventions (e.g. cognitive behavior therapy) and pharmacological approaches (e.g. clozapine).

Smoking

Cigarette smoking by patients with schizophrenia exceeds the rates in the general US population by two- to threefold (Evins et al., 2019). The prevalence of cigarette smoking in patients with schizophrenia is between 70% and 90%, compared to 35–55% for all other psychiatric patients and 30–35% for the general population. It is not entirely clear why patients with schizophrenia smoke at such high rates. Reasons suggested include a genetic basis, as a method of self-treatment, or an underlying neurobiological cause (nicotinergic deficit). Many patients start smoking after the first episode of psychosis. The nature of smoking seems to differ, as well (smoking high-tar cigarettes and for longer periods, inhaling more deeply).

Smoking offsets the sedative effects from psychotropic medications. It has been shown that smoking lowers blood levels of many psychoactive agents, including APDs, by activating hepatic enzyme systems and thereby increasing their metabolism, and may help overcome akathisia, dystonia and parkinsonism. These findings lend support to the idea of self-medication – more correctly, self-treatment of side effects. Thus, medication dosing has to be adjusted to smoking status, and in the event of sudden smoking cessation the blood levels of drugs can rise dramatically, resulting in toxicity. Dose reduction is often required in such situations.

Regardless of the reasons for high rates of smoking, it is associated with increased medical morbidity but surprisingly not for lung cancer. Patients should be referred to smoking cessation programs and coordinate closely with psychiatric care. Pharmacological aids to smoking cessation include nicotine patches and gum, bupropion, varenicline and possibly clozapine.

Summary

- Recovery is more than the absence of major symptoms. Functional recovery involves resumption of social and role functioning. Personal recovery, which involves adaptive integration of one's life goals despite the illness, can occur despite or alongside various levels of symptomatic or functional losses.
- Recovery assessment and treatment planning should be individualized. Each patient has a unique set of interacting factors that influence the extent of recovery.

- There are at least ten factors important for achieving recovery: **access to care, cognitive abilities, duration of untreated psychosis, family relationships, initial response to medication, personal history, substance abuse, social skills, supportive therapy and treatment adherence.**
- Co-morbidity can significantly impact treatment and outcome. **Depressive symptoms** are common in schizophrenia, occurring in 25–40% of patients. First-episode patients tend to have more severe depression compared with multi-episode patients. Persistent hopelessness at discharge is associated with poor outcome. Depression accompanying psychosis is seen in major depression, bipolar disorder and parkinsonism, and primary negative symptoms can be mistaken for depression. SSRIs and some atypical APDs are quite effective in treating depression in schizophrenia.
- As many as half of all patients with schizophrenia will **abuse substances** during their lifetime; the most common are nicotine and alcohol, followed by cannabis and cocaine. Substance abuse has many dire consequences and treatment is not easy. An integrated approach to assessment and treatment is required. Treatment consists of psychoeducation, motivational interviewing, cognitive behavior therapy and pharmacotherapy.
- Patients with schizophrenia in the US have high rates of cigarette smoking (70%–90%). Patients tend to smoke high-tar cigarettes and inhale more deeply. Smoking counters the sedative effects from psychotropic medications, lowers blood levels of many psychoactive agents and may help overcome extrapyramidal side effects. Smoking is associated with significant medical morbidity and patients should be referred to smoking cessation programs. Pharmacological aids against smoking include nicotine patches and gum, bupropion and possibly clozapine.

References

Evins, A. E., Cather, C., & Daumit, G. L. (2019, July). Smoking cessation in people with serious mental illness. *Lancet Psychiatry*, *6*(7), 563–564.

Kline, E. R., Ferrara, M., Li, F., D'Souza, D. C., Keshavan, M., & Srihari, V. H. (2022, March). Timing of cannabis exposure relative to prodrome and psychosis onset in a community-based first episode psychosis sample. *Journal of Psychiatric Research, 147*, 248–253.

Slade, M., Amering, M., Farkas, M., Hamilton, B., O'Hagan, M., Panther, G., Perkins, R., Shepherd, G., Tse, S., & Whitley, R. (2014, February). Uses and abuses of recovery: Implementing recovery-oriented practices in mental health systems. *World Psychiatry, 13*(1), 12–20.

chapter 16

History of schizophrenia

Texts from Egypt and Mesopotamia from the second millennium BCE, as well as the *Atharvaveda*, an ancient Indian scripture (ca. 1000 BCE), contain descriptions of serious mental illness. However, descriptions consistent with the modern conception of schizophrenia emerge in the 18th century. Some psychiatric historians suggest that schizophrenia is an ancient disorder, while others argue that it is a relatively modern one, no more than two centuries old (Jeste et al., 1985). This is more than an academic debate. If schizophrenia is indeed of recent origin, then it suggests that historically recent changes, likely environmental, may be responsible for the emergence of schizophrenia.

The history of schizophrenia is the history of keen clinical observation. Psychiatrists had the opportunity to observe the natural progression of schizophrenia over the course of years, if not the entire lifetimes of patients. This allowed careful descriptions of clinical syndromes and their natural courses. Nosology was in vogue during the 19th century, leading to a variety of systems of classification of mental disorders. Below is a glimpse of a few of the luminaries who contributed to the modern concept of schizophrenia (see Figure 16.1).

In the main, the history of the *concept* of schizophrenia is the history of keen clinical observation and classification by psychiatrists during the 19th and 20th centuries (Table 16.1).

Phillipe Pinel (1745–1826). Pinel's dictum to his students is still valid today: 'Take written notes at the sickbed and record the entire course of

DOI: 10.4324/9781315152806-16

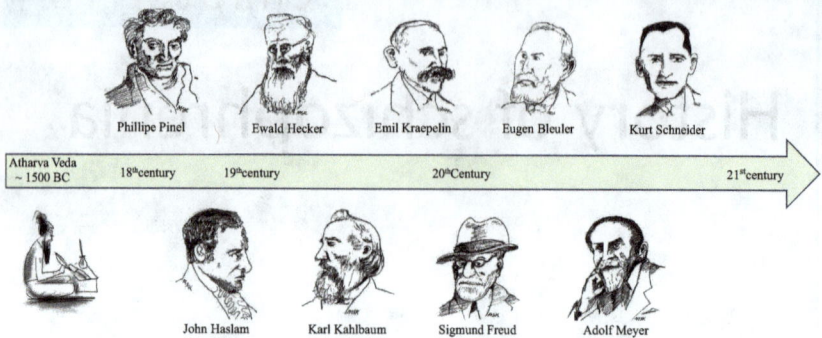

Figure 16.1 Important figures in the historical evolution of the concept of schizophrenia.

Table 16.1 Important contributions to the concept of schizophrenia

Phillipe Pinel (1745–1826)	Invented *Moral Treatment*
Benedict Morel (1809–1873)	Introduced the term *dementia praecoce*
Karl Kahlbaum (1828–1899)	Conceptualized *Katatonia*
Ewald Hecker (1843–1909)	Conceptualized *hebephrenia*
Emil Kraepelin (1856–1926)	Made the distinction between *dementia praecox* and manic-depressive psychosis
Eugen Bleuler (1857–1939)	Conceptualized and labeled *schizophrenia* with the core 'As' (autism, ambivalence, disturbances in association and affectivity)
Kurt Schneider (1887–1967)	Defined the *first-rank symptoms*
Karl Jaspers (1886–1969)	*Highlighted importance of distinguishing form vs. content when defining hallucinations and delusions*
Adolf Meyer (1866–1950)	Considered schizophrenia to be caused by harmful habits in conjunction with biological factors as well as heredity.
Sigmund Freud (1856–1939)	Introduced concepts of *projection* and primary narcissism.

severe illness'. He is considered one of the founders of psychiatry. His 'Moral Treatment' was the first attempt at individual psychotherapy. He emphasized hygiene, physical exercise and work for his patients.

John Haslam (1764–1844). In 1810, Haslam, a leading psychiatrist of the early-19th century at London's Bethlem Hospital, published a book that contains a detailed description of James Tilly Matthews' psychosis, the first clear description of schizophrenia.

Benedict Morel (1809–1873). In 1860, Morel introduced the term *dementia praecoce* to refer to a mental deterioration 'for an illness beginning in adolescence and leading to gradual deterioration'.

Karl Kahlbaum (1828–1899). Kahlbaum was the director of his own institution for the mentally ill in Görlitz, Germany. He was the first to distinguish between clinical presentations and underlying diseases. He coined the term *Katatonia* in 1868.

Ewald Hecker (1843–1909). Hecker worked with Kahlbaum in Görlitz, after which he bought his own psychiatric hospital in Wiesbaden, Germany. He was never given an academic position because of his liberal views. His classic paper on *hebephrenia* was published in 1871, in which he described a syndrome of early-onset psychosis with a deteriorating course, with 'silly' affect, behavioral oddities and thought disorder.

Emil Kraepelin (1856–1926). Undoubtedly one of the most important figures in psychiatry. In 1883, Kraepelin wrote his *Compendium der Psychiatrie*. In its sixth edition (1899), he presented the distinction between manic-depressive psychosis and dementia praecox. Kraepelin also distinguished at least three clinical varieties of dementia praecox: catatonia, hebephrenia and paranoia. Kraepelin campaigned against smoking and alcohol. In the Munich psychiatric clinic, all alcohol was banned, and patients were offered lemonade (*Kraepelinsekt*).

Eugen Bleuler (1857–1939). Bleuler coined the term 'schizophrenia' to describe a 'splitting' of mental functions. He wrote, 'I call dementia praecox "schizophrenia" because (as I hope to demonstrate) the "splitting" of the different psychic functions is one of its most important characteristics. For the sake of convenience, I use the word in the singular although it is apparent that the group includes several diseases'.

He considered certain symptoms (*Bleuler's four 'As'*: autism, ambivalence, disturbances in association and affectivity) to be 'fundamental' while others, such as delusions and hallucinations, were 'accessory' symptoms, because they were found in other disorders.

Kurt Schneider (1887–1967). Schneider identified certain types of delusions and hallucinations as being characteristic of schizophrenia ('First Rank Symptoms'). These criteria, published in 1959, represented a narrow concept of schizophrenia.

Adolf Meyer (1866–1950). Meyer is rightly known as 'the dean of American psychiatry'. He advocated a thorough understanding of the patient as a whole person. He also argued for integrating psychology and biology into a single system, psychobiology, which was to be applied to assessment and treatment, with the goal of helping the patient adjust to life and change. A component of the therapy, called 'habit training', was to help patients, including those with schizophrenia, modify unhealthy adjustments by guidance, suggestion and re-education. He considered schizophrenia to be caused by harmful habits in conjunction with biological factors as well as heredity.

Sigmund Freud (1856–1939). Freud's contributions towards understanding schizophrenia include the concepts of projection and primary narcissism. Projection is a defense mechanism, operating unconsciously, in which emotionally unacceptable impulses are rejected and attributed to others. He referred to schizophrenia as 'paraphrenia', and was doubtful that psychoanalysis could help.

In spite of the progress made during the previous century, the early and mid-20th century was marked by descriptive and diagnostic inconsistency. Further, the lack of understanding of etiopathology of the illness contributed to significant variations in the frequency of diagnosis of schizophrenia. During the 1960s, the World Health Organization (WHO) took the initiative to establish a set of criteria that gradually evolved into the International Classification of Diseases (currently in its eleventh revision, ICD-11). A multinational study conducted by the World Health Organization, using standardized criteria, revealed similar worldwide prevalence of schizophrenia. The latest diagnostic scheme, *Diagnostic and Statistical Manual*, Fifth Edition text revision (DSM-5-TR, American Psychiatric Association 2022), has incorporated several significant changes in the diagnostic criteria for schizophrenia. Although there are critiques of the validity of these diagnostic criteria, the ICD and DSM have improved diagnostic reliability and understanding of schizophrenia. Other approaches to classification of schizophrenia have included type 1 and 2 schizophrenia based on symptoms and brain structure (Crow, 1980), positive vs. negative symptom categories (Andreasen & Olsen, 1982) and deficit vs. non-deficit schizophrenia (Carpenter et al., 1988).

Further refinements in diagnosis will likely come from advancements in genetics and neurobiology. Recent efforts have focused on developing categorical classifications of psychotic disorders using biomarkers to generate biological subtypes or biotypes across primary psychotic disorders (Clementz et al., 2016). The Research Domain Criteria (RDoC) framework, developed by leading scientists and led by the National Institute of Mental Health (Insel et al., 2010), provides a dimensional framework to understand psychopathology in the context of major biological and behavioral domains, rather than within symptom-based diagnostic categories. The Hierarchical Taxonomy of Psychopathology (HiTOP) is another way of classifying psychiatric disorders, based on empirical psychopathological data as they vary dimensionally from healthy to ill populations (Kotov et al., 2022).

Summary

- The history of mental illness extends back over two millennia, recorded in early writings from Egypt, Mesopotamia and India.
- Descriptions of schizophrenia, as defined today, appear in the 18th century. The earliest description was provided by John Haslam in 1810.
- Schizophrenia may be a relatively modern disorder, suggesting that the impacts – probably environmental – of modernity may be responsible for the emergence of schizophrenia.
- The concept of schizophrenia is still evolving and is best conceptualized currently as a heterogeneous syndrome that may include multiple psychopathological dimensions and pathophysiological processes.

References

Andreasen, N. C., & Olsen, S. (1982, July). Negative v positive schizophrenia. Definition and validation. *Archives of General Psychiatry, 39*(7), 789–794.

Carpenter, W. T. Jr, Heinrichs, D. W., & Wagman, A. M. (1988, May). Deficit and nondeficit forms of schizophrenia: The concept. *American Journal of Psychiatry, 145*(5), 578–583.

Clementz, B. A., Sweeney, J. A., Hamm, J. P., Ivleva, E. I., Ethridge, L. E., Pearlson, G. D., Keshavan, M. S., & Tamminga, C. A. (2016, April 1). Identification of distinct psychosis biotypes using brain-based biomarkers. *American Journal of Psychiatry, 173*(4), 373–384.

Crow, T. J. (1980, January 12). Molecular pathology of schizophrenia: More than one disease process? *British Medical Journal, 280*(6207), 66–68.

Insel, T., Cuthbert, B., Garvey, M., Heinssen, R., Pine, D. S., Quinn, K., Sanislow, C., & Wang, P. (2010, July). Research domain criteria (RDoC): Toward a new classification framework for research on mental disorders. *American Journal of Psychiatry, 167*(7), 748–751.

Jeste, D. V., del Carmen, R., Lohr, J. B., & Wyatt, R. J. (1985, November–December). Did schizophrenia exist before the eighteenth century? *Comprehensive Psychiatry, 26*(6), 493–503.

Kotov, R., Cicero, D. C., Conway, C. C., DeYoung, C. G., Dombrovski, A., Eaton, N. R., First, M. B., Forbes, M. K., Hyman, S. E., Jonas, K. G., Krueger, R. F., Latzman, R. D., Li, J. J., Nelson, B. D., Regier, D. A., Rodriguez-Seijas, C., Ruggero, C. J., Simms, L. J., Skodol, A. E., . . . Wright, A. G. C. (2022, July). The hierarchical taxonomy of psychopathology (HiTOP) in psychiatric practice and research. *Psychological Medicine, 52*(9), 1666–1678.

chapter 17

Who gets schizophrenia and why?

In discussing who might develop schizophrenia and why that might be the case, there are genetic and epigenetic factors to consider. Since the precise pathology of schizophrenia is not known, epidemiological (Greek *epi* = upon; *demos* = people; *logos* = word, discourse; the study of occurrence of diseases in human populations) methods are used to investigate the possible determinants of schizophrenia.

Epidemiology is the study of the occurrence, distribution and determinants of schizophrenia.

Incidence is the number of newly diagnosed cases during a specific time period. In any given year, three to six individuals will be newly diagnosed with schizophrenia out of a population of 10,000 (incidence rate: 30–60 in 100,000).

Prevalence can be expressed as the number of cases of a disease present in a particular population at a particular point in time (point prevalence). Current research indicates a prevalence of four to seven per 1,000 persons. There are approximately 50 million individuals worldwide diagnosed with schizophrenia, including 2.2 million in the USA, 250,000 in Great Britain, 8.7 million in India, 12 million in China, 280,000 in Canada and 285,000 in Australia.

Lifetime prevalence is the number of individuals in the population who will develop the disorder at some point during their lifetime. Latest research indi-

DOI: 10.4324/9781315152806-17

cates that the lifetime prevalence of schizophrenia is approximately 0.5% – lower than the traditionally quoted 1%.

There are **geographical variations** in prevalence. Regions of higher prevalence (also called geographical isolates) include Croatia, some islands in Micronesia, northern Sweden and Finland and parts of Ireland. Lower prevalence is seen in Botswana, Ghana, Papua New Guinea and Taiwan.

There are also **communities** with prevalence rates higher than the region in which they are located; examples include aboriginals of Australia and natives of northern Canada. Jamaican immigrants in the UK, compared with Jamaicans in Jamaica, appear to have a higher rate of schizophrenia, which may be related to migration stress. Lower prevalence rates are seen in the Amish and Hutterite communities in the USA.

Is schizophrenia inherited?

Eugen Bleuler noted that relatives of patients with schizophrenia were often 'tainted by hereditary mental disease'. In recent years, the genetic basis of this illness has been well established. In the 1980s, psychiatrists such as Thomas Szasz held the view that schizophrenia as a disease may be a myth and that it is caused mainly by problems of living. In response, Seymour Kety famously said, 'If schizophrenia is a myth, it is a genetically transmitted myth!' It is well established that schizophrenia aggregates in families. This is the result of interactions between genetic risk and both shared and non-shared environmental factors, which can begin to act during fetal development. While the full list and precise mechanism of these *gene-environment interactions* are topics of active research, this integrative concept should replace simple contrasts between nature and nurture.

Family, twin and adoption studies have demonstrated that the chance of developing schizophrenia increases with biological proximity to the affected individual, establishing that a significant portion of risk for schizophrenia is *heritable (i.e. explained by genetic factors)*. The likelihood that an individual will develop schizophrenia increases from about 0.5% in the general population to almost 50% if both parents or an identical twin is affected, with risk estimates between the two poles varying with degree of relatedness (Figure 17.1).

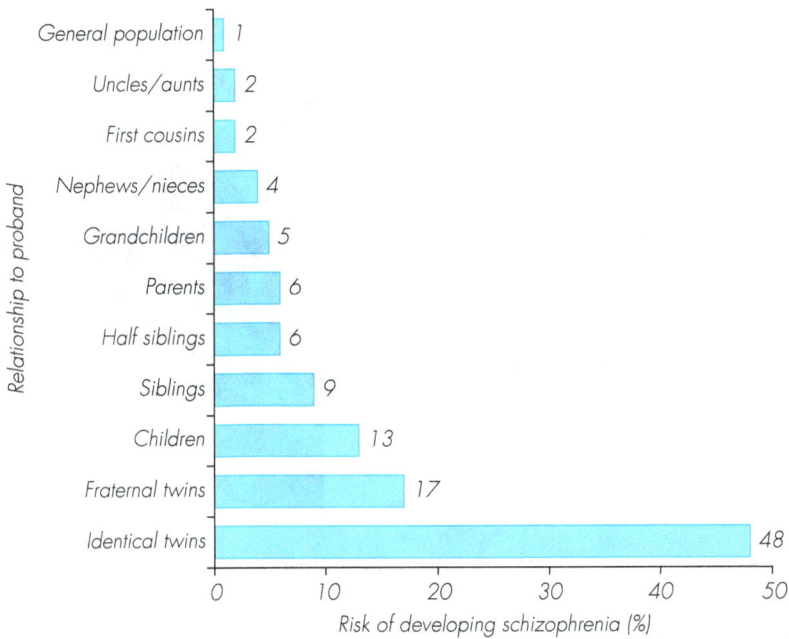

Figure 17.1 Risk of developing schizophrenia as affected by closeness of relatives with the disease.

Source: Adapted from Gottesman (1991).

How is schizophrenia transmitted?

The specific mode of transmission of schizophrenia is unclear, but several models have been proposed. Evidence to date is incompatible with either single genes or simple combinations of genes as sufficient to explain heritability. Most cases of schizophrenia likely arise from the individually small effects of a very large number of variations in DNA sequences. Also, rare cases arise from the larger effects of fewer variations in the number of longer sections of DNA (or Copy Number Variations). Further, given that many of these genetic sources of risk are in areas that regulate expression of genes, this supports the epidemiological evidence of 'epigenetic' or environmental influences on the development of schizophrenia.

Rare genes, large effect

Unknown,
Environmental
Factors.
Gene-
Environment
interactions

Common genes, small effect

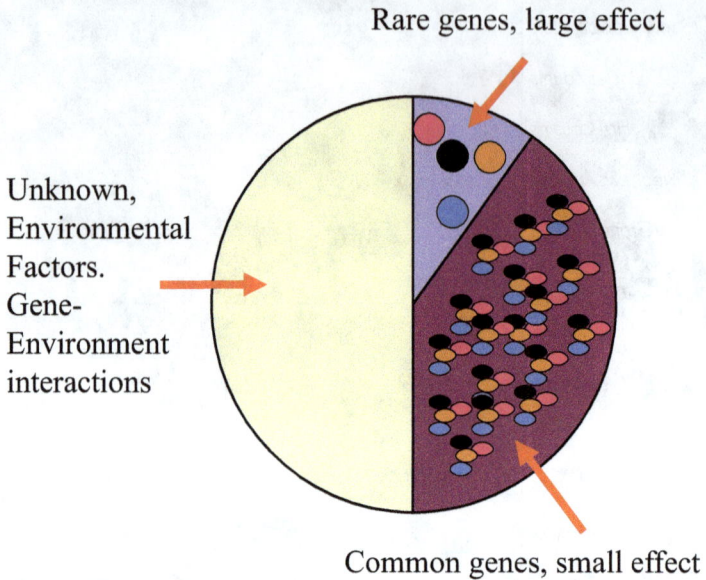

Figure 17.2 There may be multiple etiological factors in what we call schizophrenia.

What is transmitted?

Schizophrenia is a complex disorder that affects multiple domains of higher
level functioning and cannot be tied simply to genes. Rather, what may be
transmitted is a *liability* for developing the illness. This liability may express
itself as poor psychosocial functioning, unusual behavior or non-affective
psychoses. Biological relatives of individuals with schizophrenia have a
higher prevalence of schizophrenia but also schizotypal personality disorder; and these disorders have thus been considered **schizophrenia spectrum disorders.** However, unusual or idiosyncratic thinking and behavioral
disturbances are imprecise indicators of risk.

Endophenotypes (illness traits that are between the phenotype and gen-
otype), such as SPEM (Smooth Pursuit Eye Movement) dysfunction and
sustained attentional deficits (Figure 17.3), may serve as biological **vulnerability markers** and are increasingly being utilized as a detection strategy
in genetic studies.

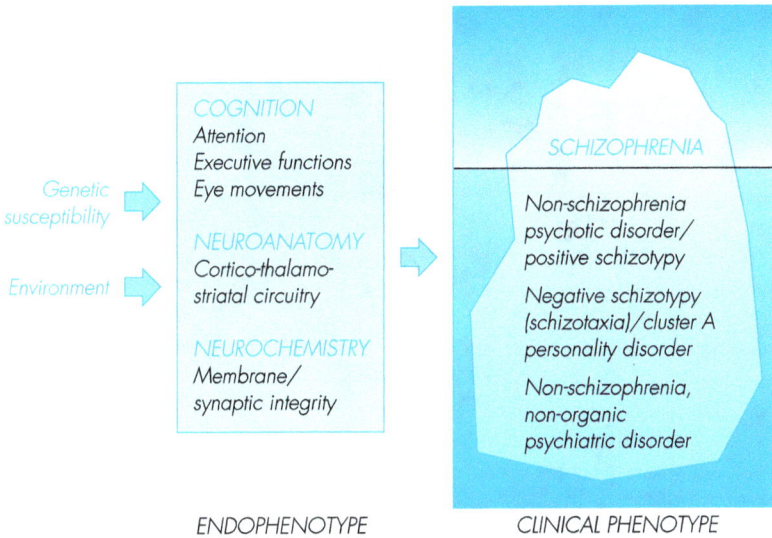

Figure 17.3 Endophenotypes are intermediate to gene/environment risk and the phenotype.

The search for schizophrenia genes

Advances in molecular genetic techniques and the recent mapping of the human genome have expanded our knowledge of risk genes in schizophrenia. The final objective of gene-hunting is to identify gene products or regulatory regions that control gene expression, which will explain the pathophysiology of schizophrenia and ultimately inform its cure.

Large genome-wide association studies (i.e. studies comparing more than 25,000 patients with a similar number of controls) have begun to identify certain genes that are associated with disease risk, particularly those that may play a role in brain development and plasticity (Schizophrenia Working Group, 2014). Recent observations suggest that immune-related genes such as complement4 may be strongly linked to the risk for schizophrenia (Sekar et al., 2016). Variations in genes such as *ZNF804A*, *DISC1*, *TCF4* and *NRGN* may confer a slightly increased risk of schizophrenia. Rare copy number variants (CNV), which are deletions or duplications of portions of the genome, such as deletions in regions 22q11.2, 1q21.1, and 17p12, are also associated with schizophrenia. Another interesting

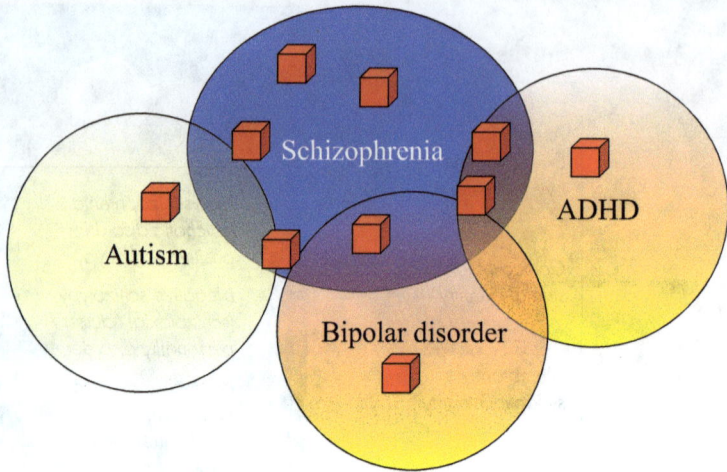

Figure 17.4 Genetic factors in schizophrenia overlap with those for bipolar disorder, autism and ADHD.

Source: Smoller (2013).

result from genetic studies is that many of the genes that confer risk for schizophrenia are associated with other neuropsychiatric disorders, such as bipolar disorder, autism and attention-deficit disorder (Smoller, 2013; see Figure 17.4).

Environmental factors and gene-environmental interactions

As noted above, genes have a prominent, but not exclusive role in the pathogenesis of schizophrenia. Studies have shown that monozygotic twin pairs, who share 100% of their genes, are not 100% concordant (i.e. if one twin has the illness, the co-twin has only a 50% chance of having the illness). This suggests that environmental influences play an important role in the development of schizophrenia. There are several environmental factors that consistently have been found to be associated with schizophrenia (Table 17.1), although the mechanism of their influence has not been deciphered. In recent years, Social Determinants of Health (SDoHs) are

Table 17.1 Environmental risk factors

Perinatal complications	History of pregnancy and birth complications (e.g. pre-eclampsia, prematurity, low birth weight) are present in about 25% of patients, more often in males. Hypoxic brain injury may be one mechanism mediating the effects of birth complications. Prenatal exposure to influenza in the second trimester and nutritional deficiencies are other environmental factors that increase the risk of schizophrenia.
Paternal age	Fathers above the age of 45 had a twofold elevated risk, and fathers above the age of 50 had a threefold elevated risk of having offspring develop schizophrenia, compared to fathers at or below the age of 25. Although the mechanisms remain unclear, accumulation of several point mutations during the replications of spermatogonial stem cells and epigenetic changes related to methylation, demethylation and histone modifications have been proposed.
Trauma	Trauma of various kinds (physical and sexual abuse, neglect) have been associated with the risk for schizophrenia. Overall, a three- to sevenfold increase in risk for schizophrenia is reported when the trauma occurred before the age of 16.
Season of birth	In the northern hemisphere, schizophrenia patients tend to be born more frequently between January and April; in the southern hemisphere, the same is true between July and September. It has been suggested that viral infections may account for this correlation.
Cannabis abuse	There is increasing evidence that heavy cannabis abuse during adolescence increases the risk for later schizophrenia (D'Souza et al., 2022). The greater the dose, and the earlier the age of exposure, the greater the risk. The liberalization of cannabis use in USA in recent years is of concern. Delaying or eliminating exposure to cannabis or cannabinoids could potentially impact the rates of psychosis related to cannabis, especially in those who are at high risk for developing the disorder.

receiving growing attention and may be particularly relevant to persons with schizophrenia (Jester et al., 2023).

Models of illness development that consider gene-environment interaction are critically important. It has become increasingly clear that several environmental factors, such as substance misuse, can modify gene expression. The study of this effect, called epigenetics, may elucidate many aspects of the causation of schizophrenia.

Summary

- Schizophrenia runs in families and has a high degree of heritability.
- Causes of schizophrenia involve a large number of genes and several environmental factors that may interact to lead to this illness.
- The causal factors of schizophrenia are not specific to this illness and overlap considerably with other disorders such as bipolar disorder, autism and neurodevelopmental disorders.

References

D'Souza, D. C., DiForti, M., Ganesh, S., George, T. P., Hall, W., Hjorthøj, C., Howes, O., Keshavan, M., Murray, R. M., Nguyen, T. B., Pearlson, G. D., Ranganathan, M., Selloni, A., Solowij, N., & Spinazzola, E. (2022, December). Consensus paper of the WFSBP task force on cannabis, cannabinoids and psychosis. *World Journal of Biological Psychiatry*, *23*(10), 719–742.

Gottesman, I. I. (1991). *Schizophrenia genesis: The origin of madness*. Freeman.

Jester, D. J., Thomas, M. L., Sturm, E. T., Harvey, P. D., Keshavan, M., Davis, B. J., Saxena, S., Tampi, R., Leutwyler, H., Compton, M. T., Palmer, B. W., & Jeste, D. V. (2023, April 6). Review of major social determinants of health in schizophrenia-spectrum psychotic disorders: I. Clinical outcomes. *Schizophrenia Bulletin*. Epub ahead of print. PMID: 37022779.

Schizophrenia Working Group. (2014). Biological insights from 108 schizophrenia-associated genetic loci. *Nature*, *511*(7510), 421–427.

Sekar, A., Bialas, A. R., de Rivera, H., Davis, A., Hammond, T. R., Kamitaki, N., Tooley, K., Presumey, J., Baum, M., Van Doren, V., Genovese, G., Rose, S. A., Handsaker, R. E., Schizophrenia Working Group of the Psychiatric Genomics Consortium, Daly, M. J., Carroll, M. C., Stevens, B., & McCarroll, S. A. (2016). Schizophrenia risk from complex variation of complement component 4. *Nature*, *530*(7589), 177–183.

Smoller, J. W. (2013). Identification of risk loci with shared effects on five major psychiatric disorders: A genome-wide analysis. *The Lancet*, *381*(9875), 1371–1379.

chapter 18

Neurobiology of schizophrenia

Schizophrenia has stubbornly resisted yielding its secrets, despite a century of research. However, much has been learned about disturbances in the brain *associated* with the disorder. Recent studies utilizing neuroimaging, neurophysiology, neurochemistry and neuropathological methods have advanced our understanding of the brain circuitry and biochemical underpinnings of schizophrenia.

Early studies largely relied on postmortem examinations of the brains of mostly older patients with chronic schizophrenia or brain scans in patients with established schizophrenia, many of whom had substantial exposure to medications. It was difficult, therefore, to tease apart the effects of the illness from those of aging, illness chronicity and medications. Studies of individuals in the early phases of schizophrenia, especially those in the first episode, have advanced our understanding considerably.

Neuroanatomical alterations

Over a quarter-century ago, computed tomography (CT) showed that patients with schizophrenia have a reduction in brain tissue, as evidenced by enlarged cerebral ventricles (Figure 18.1). Several magnetic resonance imaging (MRI) studies have confirmed significant abnormalities in brain structure in patients with schizophrenia and firmly established a neurobiological basis for schizophrenia.

DOI: 10.4324/9781315152806-18

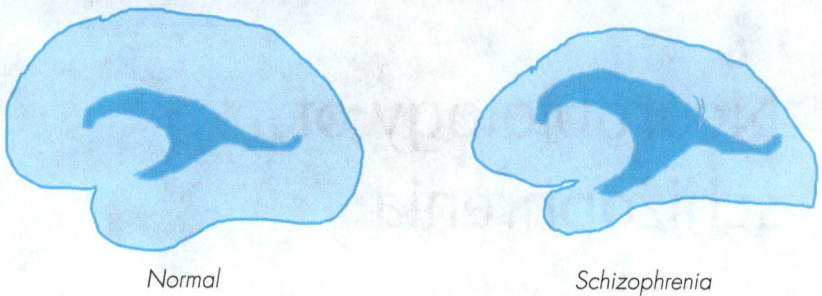

Normal   Schizophrenia

Figure 18.1 Enlarged cerebral ventricles and cortical thinning.

It has been known since the early part of the 20th century that schizophrenia patients frequently show enlargement of the cerebral ventricles, as shown in pneumoencephalographic studies. The advent of CT scanning in the 1970s confirmed the observations that lateral ventricles are enlarged in a substantial proportion of schizophrenic patients; these data were replicated with subsequent MRI studies (Figure 18.2).

MRI research has delineated the following structural brain abnormalities:

- reduced brain volume of about 5–10%, with reductions especially in gray matter
- enlarged lateral and third ventricles
- decreased volumes of the prefrontal, superior temporal and medial temporal cortex, notably the hippocampus, and amygdala
- reductions in volumes of subcortical structures such as cerebellar, caudate and thalamic volumes
- white matter alterations, including reductions in the size of the corpus callosum
- reversal or loss of the asymmetry of the cerebral hemispheres

Neuroanatomical alterations appear to be present at the onset of the illness. Alterations are seen in gray matter as well as white matter. Whether these abnormalities are **static or progressive** has been an important question. Static 'lesions' would suggest that the pathological 'event' has already occurred in the past and thus may not be reversible. On the other hand, if brain alterations are progressive, it is suggestive of an ongoing pathological

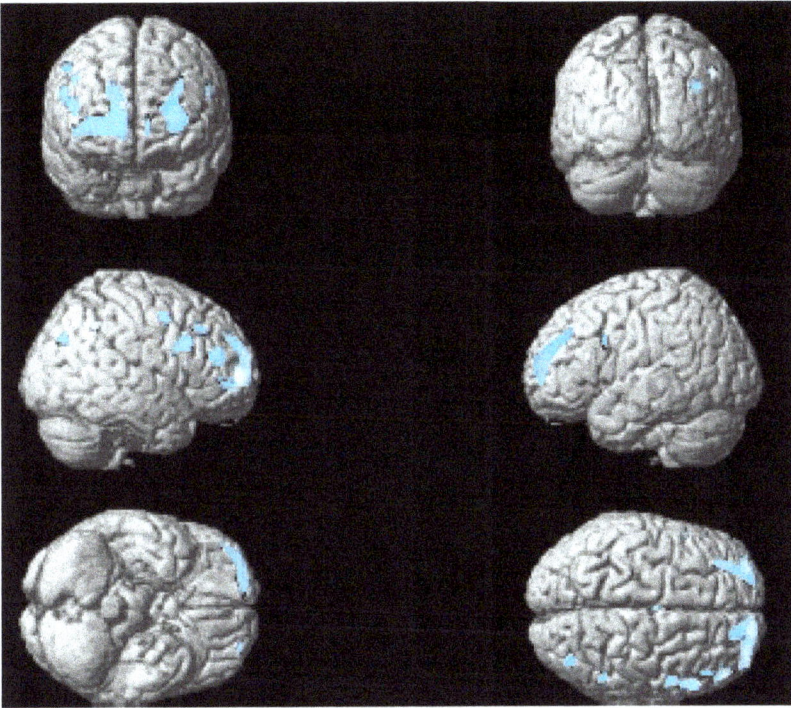

Figure 18.2 Structural brain abnormalities in schizophrenia. Brain regions with gray-matter volume reductions are shown as shaded areas.

process possibly amenable to treatment. Some studies have observed a relationship between prolonged duration of untreated psychosis and gray matter loss. First-episode patients also have less prominent structural brain abnormalities than chronically ill patients. Prospective follow-up studies of first-episode patients suggest continued gray matter loss during the first few years of the illness. Based on such findings, it has been argued that psychosis may be 'toxic' to the brain. If true, early intervention could halt the progression of brain abnormalities in schizophrenia and related psychoses, and this may translate into favorable clinical outcomes.

Since the first episode of schizophrenia is frequently preceded by subtle psychotic-like symptoms and social withdrawal (the prodromal or 'clinical high risk' phase), one wonders whether the structural brain changes may emerge in parallel to the functional decline that characterizes this period.

Individuals at high genetic risk for developing psychosis have structural alterations such as amygdala-hippocampal and thalamic volume reductions. Prospective studies have shown that high-risk individuals who later became psychotic have less gray matter in a variety of brain regions (right medial temporal, lateral temporal, inferior frontal cortex and cingulate cortex bilaterally). This is very suggestive of an active disease process taking place during the transition to psychosis.

Brain network alterations

Using techniques such as diffusion tensor imaging and resting-state and task-related functional imaging, it has been shown in recent years that schizophrenia is characterized by alterations in connectivity between widespread brain structures. Alterations in executive, reward, salience and language brain networks may underlie respectively the cognitive, negative and positive symptoms and thought disorder in this illness.

Neurochemical alterations

The conventional teaching over the past decades has been that psychotic symptoms are related to excess of dopamine. Supporting this view is the fact that all effective antipsychotics block dopamine (Figure 18.3), and the fact that agents that increase dopamine levels, such as amphetamine and cocaine, can cause psychotic symptoms. Also, there is indirect support based on observations of increased levels of homovanillic acid, a dopamine metabolite, in the cerebrospinal fluid of schizophrenic patients. Postmortem studies of dopamine receptor density have yielded inconsistent results. Recent positron emission tomography (PET) studies, however, support presynaptic alterations of dopamine transmission in schizophrenia.

A more nuanced view of the role of dopamine suggests that negative and cognitive symptoms in schizophrenia may be related to reduced activity in the mesocortical dopamine system, while positive symptoms may be related to a *hyper*dopaminergic state in the mesolimbic dopamine system (Weinberger, 1987). The mesolimbic system is normally inhibited by the mesocortical dopamine system; thus, the mesolimbic over-activity

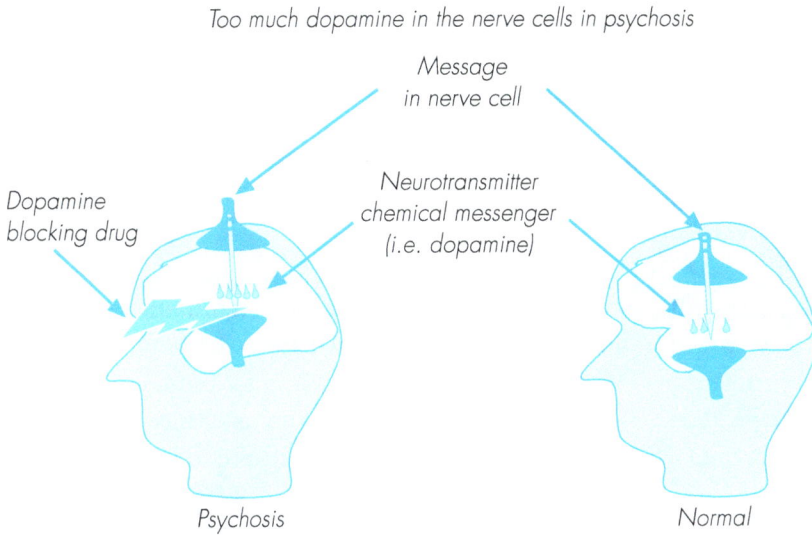

Too much dopamine in the nerve cells in psychosis

Message in nerve cell

Dopamine blocking drug

Neurotransmitter chemical messenger (i.e. dopamine)

Psychosis

Normal

Figure 18.3 The classical **dopamine excess theory** of schizophrenia. It is generally believed that psychosis is related to an excess of neurotransmitter release by the dopaminergic neurons (left) in comparison with healthy persons (right). This view is consistent with the observation that all antipsychotic drugs have an effect of blocking one or other type of dopamine receptor to a greater or lesser extent.

may be due to disinhibition from the cortical 'brakes'. The most recent articulation of a modified dopamine hypothesis sees hyperdopaminergia in the mesolimbic system as explaining only the positive symptoms of the psychosis syndrome. While this makes for a more modest account of the illness, it remains the most applicable in medication choice and also offers a useful way to describe or at least speculate about how this abnormality can lead to a subjective sense of 'aberrant salience' in the patient. This can offer patients and families a way to appreciate that odd or delusional beliefs and disorganized behavior can be the result of an illness process rather than a willed choice or personality trait (Howes & Kapur, 2009).

A variety of other neurotransmitters are likely involved in the pathogenesis of schizophrenia. It is also possible that more fundamental defects, perhaps in cellular membranes, may be implicated. For each of these alternative hypotheses, varying degrees of evidence are available.

Glutamate

Glutamate, an excitatory neurotransmitter, is the most abundant neurotransmitter. Phencyclidine, a glutamatergic receptor antagonist, causes symptoms similar to schizophrenia. Post-mortem studies have suggested that brains of individuals with schizophrenia may have alterations in glutamatergic receptors.

Gamma-Amino Butyric Acid (GABA)

Loss of GABA interneurons, an inhibitory neurotransmitter, has been observed in the hippocampus and the cingulate in schizophrenia. Such impairment in GABA inhibitory inputs could lead to disinhibited activity of the glutamatergic system and, consequently, an imbalance in the mesocortical and mesolimbic dopamine systems, as reflected in Figure 18.4.

Other neurotransmitter systems

A potential role of serotonin (5-hydroxytryptamine, 5-HT) in schizophrenia has been suggested. Lysergic acid diethylamide (LSD), a drug with strong serotonin effects, can cause psychosis. Drugs such as clozapine that block

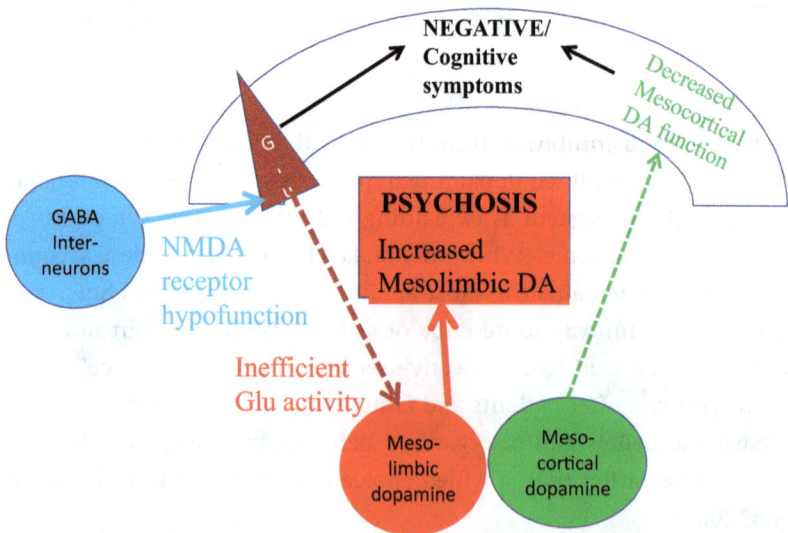

Figure 18.4 The current conceptualization of the neurochemical 'imbalance' in schizophrenia.

5-HT as well as dopamine are highly effective for schizophrenia. Another neurotransmitter implicated in schizophrenia is acetylcholine. In recent years, some medications are being developed to treat schizophrenia that target the cholinergic system (see chapter 19).

Neurophysiological alterations

Electrophysiological studies use the electroencephalogram (EEG), a recording of the brain's electrical activity over time, to study neurobiological changes in schizophrenia. Most of these studies present specific sequences of auditory stimuli to patients and measure event-related potentials, which are the electrophysiological responses to the stimuli. Types of event-related potential markers, such as the mismatch negativity, P50, N100 and P300, vary in the timing and sequence of auditory or visual stimuli. Individuals with schizophrenia differ from healthy controls in the waveform characteristics of these markers. Many electrophysiological markers are also abnormal in the relatives of patients with schizophrenia, indicating hereditary influence. The clinical significance of these markers is still being worked out, but some of them correlate with cognitive function and may represent aspects of early information processing.

Neuropathological evidence

While 19th-century studies failed to find any abnormalities in postmortem brains of schizophrenia patients, studies over the last decades have revealed subtle reductions in cerebral volume and thinning of the cerebral cortex, selective reductions in the volume of the thalamus and reductions in medial temporal cortical volume.

Histopathological studies have revealed reduced neuronal size, reduced dendritic density, decreased concentrations of synaptic proteins such as synaptophysins and possible increased neuronal packing density (see Figure 18.5). These findings have suggested the possibility that in schizophrenia there are reductions in synaptic neuropil, perhaps related to the processes of exaggerated synaptic pruning that happen normally during adolescence.

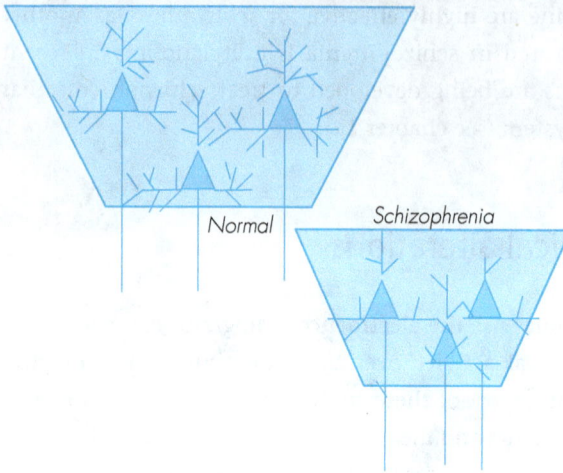

Figure 18.5 Neuronal density and decreased synapse density in schizophrenia.

When might the illness really begin?

Clarifying when schizophrenia begins will be essential to instituting appropriate early interventions to mitigate its severity or even prevent its clinical emergence. Which neurodevelopmental model best explains the progression of the disorder is a vital question.

One view, the so-called early developmental model (Weinberger, 1987), suggests that abnormalities in brain development around or before birth mediate the failure of brain functions in early adulthood. This model is supported by an array of data, such as an increased rate of birth complications, minor physical abnormalities, neurological soft signs and subtle behavioral abnormalities in children who later developed schizophrenia. However, only a small number of people with such risk indicators eventually develop schizophrenia.

An alternative view, suggested by the fact that the illness does not typically present until adolescence or early adulthood, points to a possible developmental problem around this period. Normally, adolescence is characterized by a refinement of neuronal connections leading to an elimination (or 'pruning') of surplus synapses. If this process is excessive, then a pronounced loss of synapses, perhaps of the glutamatergic

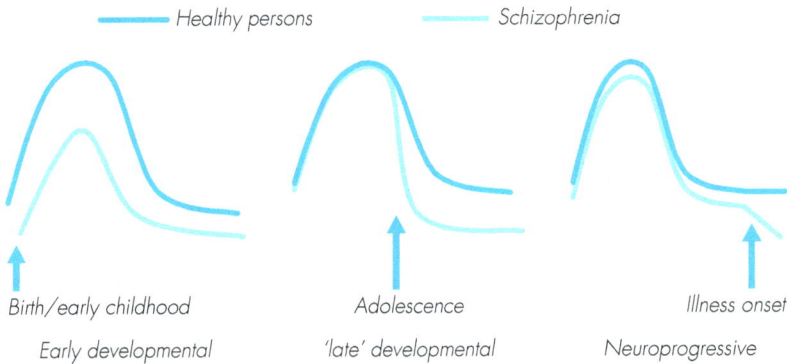

Figure 18.6 Pathophysiological models of schizophrenia.

system, may result, leading to the emergence of the illness (Feinberg, 1982/1983).

Finally, the observation that at least a subgroup of patients deteriorates over the first few years of the illness has led to the view that there may be a progressive process of neuronal or synapse loss (Stone et al., 2022).

These pathophysiological models (Figure 18.6) are not necessarily mutually exclusive. It is possible that schizophrenia is heterogeneous, i.e. there may be subgroups that differ in the nature of pathophysiology. A sequential combination of these processes is also possible, with early developmental, late developmental and neuroprogressive processes occurring in the same individual; such a 'three hit' model points to the possibility of therapeutic interventions at multiple time points in individuals at risk for schizophrenia (Keshavan, 1999). Environmental factors such as trauma, illicit drug use and psychosocial stress may also be potential secondary triggers accompanying the onset and course of schizophrenia.

Are brain changes specific to schizophrenia?

Over the past several decades it has become clear that the structural, functional and neurochemical brain alterations outlined above are not specific to schizophrenia, but are seen to varying extent across other disorders, such as schizoaffective and bipolar disorders.

Summary

- Schizophrenia is associated with widespread structural and physiological alterations, resulting in abnormal connectivity across multiple brain networks.
- Dopamine is proximately involved, but imbalances in glutamate, GABA and other molecules underlying synapse function and brain development are involved as well.
- Schizophrenia may result from synaptic pruning during adolescence and a deficit in brain plasticity.
- Brain abnormalities in psychotic disorders may cut across symptom-based diagnoses and may identify distinct biological subtypes of psychotic illness with distinct treatment targets.

References

Feinberg, I. (1982/1983). Schizophrenia: Caused by a fault in programmed synaptic elimination during adolescence? *Journal of Psychiatric Research, 17*(4), 319–334.

Howes, O. D., & Kapur, S. (2009, May). The dopamine hypothesis of schizophrenia: Version III-the final common pathway. *Schizophrenia Bulletin, 35*(3), 549–562.

Keshavan, M. S. (1999, November–December). Development, disease and degeneration in schizophrenia: A unitary pathophysiological model. *Journal of Psychiatric Research, 33*(6), 513–521.

Stone, W. S., Phillips, M. R., Yang, L. H., Kegeles, L. S., Susser, E. S., & Lieberman, J. A. (2022, May). Neurodegenerative model of schizophrenia: Growing evidence to support a revisit. *Schizophrenia Research, 243,* 154–162.

Weinberger, D. R. (1987, July). Implications of normal brain development for the pathogenesis of schizophrenia. *Archives of General Psychiatry, 44*(7), 660–669.

chapter 19

What does the future hold?

Our task in the present is to do the best we can for our patients and their families. The future, judging from the recent past, looks hopeful. It is important to maintain an optimistic outlook, for there is good cause. There continue to be advancements on many fronts – molecular genetics, integrative biology, refined psychosocial interventions, functional brain imaging, services research, complementary medicine, prevention studies and cross-national studies, to name but a few areas. First, advances in our understanding of the neurobiological features of the illness may enable development of biomarkers of value for diagnosis, treatment choice and outcome prediction. Second, neuroimaging studies have enabled identification of specific neural circuitry changes that may underlie alterations in several psychopathological domains. Finally, a better understanding of neurochemical underpinnings of schizophrenia and related illnesses points to several potential therapeutic targets for psychopharmacological treatments. These advancements will eventually translate into better-targeted, more-effective and safer treatments.

Biomarkers

There are relatively few biomarkers in clinical use in psychiatry at this time, but this is an area of active research (Abi-Dargham et al., 2023). In the area of schizophrenia, biomarkers may be of value in four settings.

DOI: 10.4324/9781315152806-19

A) *Diagnosis:* Most biomarkers overlap considerably between psychiatric disorders and are, at this time, of relatively limited diagnostic value. This may at least in part be related to the limitations of current classification of psychiatric disorders, which is primarily symptom-based (Kapur et al., 2012). Recent approaches classify psychotic disorders based on biomarker signatures into biological subtypes, or biotypes (such as electroencephalography and event-related potentials, cognition and eye-tracking measures), suggesting the possibility that such categories may be distinguishable using imaging biomarkers (Guimond et al., 2021).

B) *Susceptibility biomarkers:* An exciting development is the role of biomarkers for prediction of conversion to psychosis among individuals at clinical high risk of developing psychotic illness. Multimodal algorithms and calculators using clinical information and incorporating structural imaging data have proved helpful in predicting psychosis and are under development.

C) *Treatment-response prediction*: Biomarkers may be of value for treatment-response prediction; one example is striatal resting-state functional magnetic resonance imaging (fMRI). Striatal connectivity index (SCI) and the functional striatal abnormalities (FSA) index have been shown to be of value for prediction of treatment response in schizophrenia (Sarpal et al., 2016).

D) *Safety biomarkers*: An example is the use of pharmacogenetic biomarkers to predict adverse side effects of clozapine. Recent findings suggest that a HLA-based pharmacogenomic test may be promising for predicting agranulocytosis with clozapine (Islam et al., 2022).

For biomarkers to be actionable, they need to be independently replicated, their predictive value needs to be demonstrable at the individual level and they should be feasible in clinical settings. Given the complexity of psychiatric disorders such as schizophrenia, any single biomarker may be of limited value, and multivariate analyses of imaging, physiological and blood-based biomarkers may be needed.

Circuitry modification using neuromodulation and neurofeedback

Increasing evidence that alterations in neural connectivity underlie specific symptom domains in schizophrenia has motivated development of novel, noninvasive interventions to modify these circuits. For example, altered cerebello-frontal circuits may underlie negative symptoms, and stimulation of such circuits with transcranial magnetic stimulation may reverse such deficits (Brady et al., 2019). Similar interventions will likely be developed in the near future for other symptom domains such as hallucinations, thought disorder and cognitive deficits.

Recent technical advances in imaging and computational neuroscience have motivated interest in neurofeedback, a form of self-regulation or neuromodulation, in treatment of cognitive impairments and symptoms in schizophrenia. Patients are provided feedback on specific neural events (via visual or auditory representations of a patient's own brain activity, e.g. brain response to specific tasks as targets). Patients can practice modulating their own neural activity and thereby alleviating their symptoms. Early studies suggest that this approach is feasible (Gandara et al., 2020), but more systematic work is needed.

Novel drug development

The history of psychopharmacological treatments has largely been one of serendipity. The future, however, will likely also include interventions developed from knowledge of illness mechanisms. It is now possible to screen thousands of molecules to identify a handful that have the possibility of becoming viable treatments. Regardless of whether a drug is devised or discovered, there are processes by which safety, tolerability and efficacy have to be established prior to releasing it for general use. In the USA, the Federal Drug Administration (FDA) regulates this process.

All drugs go through a set of rigorously conducted studies. The first stage includes preclinical studies in the laboratory to comprehensively assess safety and biological activity of the test drug; this process can take three to four years. The next stage includes a series of clinical trials (phases) that can last six years or more.

Phase I trials are conducted in small groups of people (20–80) to assess safety, dosage range and possible side effects.

Phase II trials are larger studies (100–300 individuals) to assess efficacy and safety.

Phase III trials are large-scale (up to 3000 individuals) and frequently multi-site studies to confirm efficacy, compare with placebo or standard treatments and monitor safety.

After the completion of the trials, the data is submitted to the FDA. After much deliberation about the drug's safety, efficacy, risk-benefit ratio, manufacturing methods and so on, the FDA may decide to approve the drug or request additional data. Once approved (which may take up to 12 years from the initial chemical identification), marketing can begin. There are **phase IV** trials for some drugs to continue evaluating effectiveness and safety. The success rate of getting a potential drug off a laboratory shelf into a patient's hands is quite low. It is estimated that for every 5,000 compounds screened, five make it to clinical trials, and one gets approved (1:5000 = 0.02% chance of success)!

There are a number of promising compounds in the pipeline, some taking the well-trodden path of 5-hydroxytryptamine (5-HT)/dopamine (DA) antagonism, while others have novel mechanisms of action. Table 19.1 is a partial listing of some compounds at various stages of testing (see Keshavan et al., 2017 for a detailed review).

Towards precision psychiatry

There is increasing focus on moving toward precision medicine, an innovative approach to tailoring disease prevention and treatment that considers differences in individual genes, environments and lifestyles. Precision medicine is best thought of as providing the right treatment for the right patient at the right time. In order to accomplish this, precise cause(s) of the illness needs to be identified in a specific patient (like a needle in a haystack, see Figure 19.1). The current approach in treating psychotic disorders, as in rest of psychiatry, tends to be a 'one-size-fits-all' strategy, in which treatments are designed for the 'average' individual with a given diagnosis, and relatively less consideration is given to individual differences (the whole haystack). Thus, all patients with psychosis receive antipsychotic medications, analogous to treating all people with chest pain with an analgesic.

Table 19.1 Some drugs in development

Compound	Mechanism of action
Bifeprunox	Partial DA agonist/antagonist; 5-HT agonist
D-Serine	Stimulates NMDA receptors
Galantamine	Enhances cholinergic function
Glycine	Stimulates NMDA receptors
D-Amino Acid Oxidase Inhibitor	Prolongs activity of D-serine at NMDA receptors
Lamotrigine	Sodium channel blocker
Memantine	NMDA receptor antagonist
Modafinil	Increases dopamine levels in the pre-frontal cortex
Seromycin/d-cycloserine	Partial NMDA receptor agonist
Roluperidone	5-HT2A and Sigma-2 Receptor Antagonist
TAAR 1 agonist (EP-363856)	Trace amine receptor agonist
Talnetant	Neurokinin-3 antagonist
Xanomeline/Trospium	Muscarinic M1/M4 agonist with a peripheral anticholinergic agent

NMDA = N-methyl-D-aspartate; AMPA = a-amino-3-hydroxy-5-methyl-4-isoxazole propionic acid

With advanced understanding of the neurobiology of psychotic disorders, the possibility of precision medicine is a realistic goal. However, etiological heterogeneity and multifactorial causation make precision psychiatry harder to develop and implement. One approach, in the meantime, is to stratify psychotic disorders into biologically *homogeneous* subgroups that may respond differentially to treatments. Thus, if it is not possible to identify the needle in a haystack, one may begin identifying 'all sharp objects' in the haystack as a first step (Figure 19.1). One example of this 'stratified medicine' is the classification of psychoses into biological subtypes, as discussed earlier, and the testing of distinct interventions informed by the pathophysiological targets (Keshavan & Clementz, 2023).

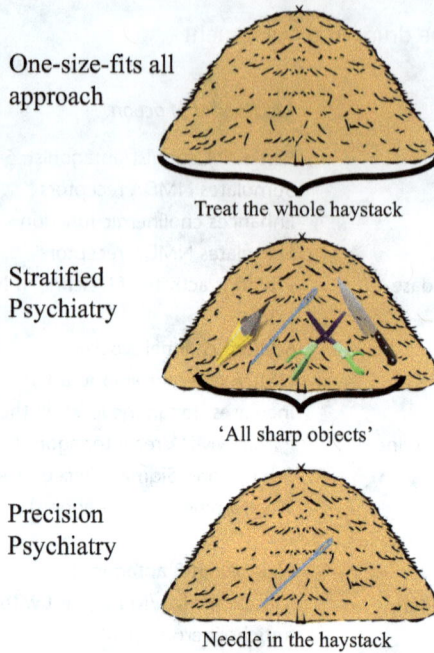

One-size-fits all
approach

Treat the whole haystack

Stratified
Psychiatry

'All sharp objects'

Precision
Psychiatry

Needle in the haystack

Figure 19.1 Toward precision psychiatry in psychotic disorders.

Services research

The application of best practices to improve outcomes for patients (*Doing what we know*) will require continued attention to the financing, regulation and management of services in a manner that facilitates both access and high-quality care for schizophrenia spectrum disorders. This effort will require continued innovation that is suited to the realities of different political-economic structures in different countries. Also, services should participate in the testing of emerging knowledge in individual patients (clinical research) and across models of care (services research). The services of the future will thus need to participate in knowledge generation (*Knowing what to do*) by both testing and generating questions for research. Traditional divisions between clinical or care-delivery workflows and research or discovery-oriented workflows will need to be weakened to allow for services that are oriented around this bi-directional mission of knowledge translation (Srihari & Cahill, 2020).

References

Abi-Dargham, A., Moeller, S. J., Ali, F., DeLorenzo, C., Domschke, K., Horga, G., Jutla, A., Kotov, R., Paulus, M. P., Rubio, J. M., Sanacora, G., Veenstra-VanderWeele, J., & Krystal, J. H. (2023, June). Candidate biomarkers in psychiatric disorders: State of the field. *World Psychiatry*, *22*(2), 236–262.

Brady, R. O. Jr, Gonsalvez, I., Lee, I., Öngür, D., Seidman, L. J., Schmahmann, J. D., Eack, S. M., Keshavan, M. S., Pascual-Leone, A., & Halko, M. A. (2019, July 1). Cerebellar-prefrontal network connectivity and negative symptoms in schizophrenia. *American Journal of Psychiatry*, *176*(7), 512–520.

Gandara, V., Pineda, J. A., Shu, I. W., & Singh, F. (2020, January). A systematic review of the potential use of neurofeedback in patients with schizophrenia. *Schizophrenia Bulletin Open*, *1*(1).

Guimond, S., Gu, F., Shannon, H., Kelly, S., Mike, L., Devenyi, G. A., Chakravarty, M. M., Sweeney, J. A., Pearlson, G., Clementz, B. A., Tamminga, C., & Keshavan, M. (2021, October 21). A diagnosis and biotype comparison across the psychosis spectrum: Investigating volume and shape amygdala-hippocampal differences from the B-SNIP study. *Schizophrenia Bulletin*, *47*(6), 1706–1717.

Islam, F., Hain, D., Lewis, D., Law, R., Brown, L. C., Tanner, J. A., & Müller, D. J. (2022, July). Pharmacogenomics of Clozapine-induced agranulocytosis: A systematic review and meta-analysis. *Pharmacogenomics Journal*, *22*(4), 230–240.

Kapur, S., Phillips, A. G., & Insel, T. R. (2012, December). Why has it taken so long for biological psychiatry to develop clinical tests and what to do about it? *Molecular Psychiatry*, *17*(12), 1174–1179.

Keshavan, M. S., & Clementz, B. A. (2023, April). Precision medicine for psychosis: A revolution at the interface of psychiatry and neurology. *Nature Reviews Neurology*, *19*(4), 193–194.

Keshavan, M. S., Lawler, A. N., Nasrallah, H. A., & Tandon, R. (2017, May). New drug developments in psychosis: Challenges, opportunities and strategies. *Progress in Neurobiology*, *152*, 3–20.

Sarpal, D. K., Argyelan, M., Robinson, D. G., Szeszko, P. R., Karlsgodt, K. H., John, M., Weissman, N., Gallego, J. A., Kane, J. M., Lencz, T., & Malhotra, A. K. (2016). Baseline striatal functional connectivity as a predictor of response to antipsychotic drug treatment. *American Journal of Psychiatry,* *173,* 69–77.

Srihari, V. H., & Cahill, J. D. Early Intervention for schizophrenia. In P. J. Uhl-haas & S. J. Wood (Eds.), *Youth mental health: A paradigm for prevention and early intervention, 2020. Strüngmann forum reports* (Vol. 28, pp. 191–208), Julia R. Lupp, series editor. MIT Press. ISBN 978-0-262-04397-7.

Glossary of terms

When there are several meanings of words, as is often the case, we have chosen the ones that are relevant to the topic at hand, namely schizophrenia.

Acting out	Expressing emotional conflict or stress through behavior and actions without reflection or regard for (usually negative) consequences.
Affect	Observable behavior that reflects the experienced emotion.
Affective blunting	AKA blunted affect. Significant reduction in affective expression.
Agranulocytosis	Granulocyte count below 500/mm³.
Akathisia	Subjective feeling of motor restlessness (jitteriness) felt mostly in the legs, often accompanied by inability to sit still or lie quietly.
Allele	One or more alternative forms of the same gene occupying a given position (locus) on a chromosome. Each person inherits two alleles for each gene, one from each parent.
Alogia	Speech that is characterized by brief and simple responses and little spontaneous speech; also called 'poverty of speech'.

Anorgasmia	Inability to achieve orgasm, even with adequate stimulation.
Association (genetics)	The relationship between specific alleles and illness in unrelated individuals (contrast with linkage). If the frequency of the specific allele in the disease population is greater than in the unrelated control population, the allele is *in association* with the disease.
Athetosis	Recurrent stream of slow, writhing movements, typically of the hands and feet; one of the movement types seen in tardive dyskinesia.
Attention	A cognitive process of selectively concentrating on one thing in a sustained manner while ignoring other stimuli. Impaired attention leads to distractibility.
Autistic thinking	Morbid self-absorption with fantastic thinking without regard to reality; one of Bleuler's 'Four As'.
Body mass index (BMI)	A measure of body fat (weight in kilograms divided by square of height in meters). BMI between 25 and 30 is defined as overweight; 30 or more is considered obese.
Capgras syndrome	Characterized by the belief that they themselves, or persons or animals of emotional significance, reflected in a mirror are impostors. Rarely, this belief extends to inanimate objects. Named after the French psychiatrist Jean Marie Joseph Capgras (1873–1950).
Catatonia	Greek *katatonos*, stretching tight. Motor abnormalities include catatonic stupor (a general absence of motor activity) and catatonic excitement

	(violent, hyperactive behavior directed at oneself or others, but with no visible purpose).
Chorea	Greek *khoreia*, choral dance. Involuntary irregular, abrupt, rapid movements involving limbs, face and trunk, that can result in lurching gait (hence, 'dancelike').
Circumstantiality	Speech pattern characterized by understandable but digressive speech with irrelevant details that delays, but does not prevent, reaching its goal.
Closed-ended question	Closed-ended questions limit responses to a pre-existing set of dichotomous answers (*Did you watch TV last night?*) or can be answered in a few words. These questions can be presuming, probing or leading.
Cognition	Latin *cognitus*, to learn, from *gno*, Indo-European roots; a broad term referring to mental processes of knowing, including aspects such as awareness, perception, reasoning and judgment.
Cotard's delusion	Characterized by the nihilistic delusion that the person is dead or does not exist. Named after Jules Cotard (1840–1889), a French neurologist.
CT	Computed tomography (CT) or computerized axial tomography (CAT) creates an image by using an array of individual X-ray sensors that spin around the patient, permitting data from multiple angles. A computer processes this information to create an image.
Culture	The totality of socially transmitted behavior patterns, arts, beliefs,

	institutions and all other products of human work and thought.
Cytochrome P450	A family of enzymes, primarily in the liver, responsible for phase I (oxidative) metabolism of drugs. Of the 40–50 isozymes, A2, 2C9, 2C19, 2D6, 3A3 and 3A4 are responsible for the metabolism of a majority of psychotropic drugs, particularly 2D6 and 3A4.
Declarative memory	The component of memory that stores facts and events. This type of information is easily forgotten and requires repetition for long-term retention.
Decompensation	Clinical worsening from current level of stability that does not meet criteria for relapse and is transitory and fluid. The clinical worsening can spontaneously return to previous level of stability without active intervention or progress to a relapsed state.
Delirium	A reversible altered state of consciousness, characterized by confusion, disorientation, disordered thinking and memory, defective perception, prominent hyperactivity, agitation and autonomic nervous system alterations. The DSM has specific diagnostic criteria.
Delusion	A fixed, false belief that is held in spite of evidence to the contrary, is at odds with the community's cultural and religious beliefs, is inconsistent with the level of education of the patient and can be patently absurd.
Dementia	Latin *demens*, senseless; dementia is characterized by loss of memory, confusion and problems with understanding, and is often associated with changes in

	personality and behavior. The DSM has specific diagnostic criteria.
Dendrites	Greek and Indo-European roots, *deru*, tree; short, highly branched fibers that carry signals *toward* the cell body of a neuron.
Denial	Defense mechanism by which unpleasant internal or external realities are kept out of conscious awareness, thus avoiding anxiety.
Derailment	AKA loosening of associations. It is a pattern of speech characterized by ideas moving from one to another in an unrelated manner. The shifts in topics are idiosyncratic.
Dermatoglyphics	The study of the skin ridges on fingertips, palms of the hands and soles of the feet. These have been used as 'archeological' evidence of developmental events *in utero* in the case of developmental disorders, including schizophrenia.
Disease	A condition in which the functioning of the body or a part of the body is interfered with or damaged. In a person with an infectious disease, the infectious agent that has entered the body causes it to function abnormally in some way or ways. The type of abnormal functioning that occurs is the disease. Usually, the body will show some signs and symptoms of the problems it is having with functioning. Disease should not be confused with infection (from Centers of Disease Control).
Disorder	Any deviation from the normal structure or function of any part, organ or

	system of the body that is manifested by a characteristic set of symptoms and signs, the pathology and prognosis of which may be known or unknown (from Centers of Disease Control).
Dominant	An allele that dominates or masks another allele when two different forms are present. Dominant alleles are represented by capital letters (e.g. Aa).
Double-bind theory	An outdated theory by Gregory Bateson about the origin of schizophrenia symptoms; they are thought to be the expression of social interactions characterized by repeated exposure to conflicting messages (usually, affection on the verbal level and animosity on the nonverbal level), without the opportunity to 'escape' from them.
Double-blind trial	A type of (clinical) trial in which neither the volunteer nor the investigator knows what treatment the volunteer is receiving, in order to minimize bias.
Downward drift hypothesis	A theory that attempts to provide a sociocultural basis for schizophrenia. This theory basically states that, given the level of functional impairment that occurs and is necessary for diagnosis, this impairment will also occur in functional and occupational areas of life and lead to a downward drift in socioeconomic status.
Dyskinesia	Abnormal involuntary movements, including athetosis and chorea.
Dysphoria	A feeling of unpleasantness, unease and emotional discomfort.
Dystonia	Acute muscular spasms, particularly of the tongue, jaw, eyes and neck, and sometimes of the whole body.

Echolalia	Greek *lalia*, speech. Senseless repetition (echoing) of words or phrases of others, immediately after their utterance or later.
Echopraxia	Greek *praxis*, action. Senseless imitating or mirroring (echoing) the movements of others.
Effectiveness	The measure of a desired result from an intervention under usual clinical conditions. In other words, does the treatment work when used under ordinary circumstances?
Efficacy	The measure of a specific desired effect resulting from an intervention, usually under ideal experimental conditions (not the same as effectiveness).
Emotion	Latin *movere*, to move. Expression of spontaneously arising internal states of being, often associated with physiological changes. Basic emotions include anger, disgust, fear, joy, sadness and surprise. However, there is little consensus regarding what constitutes basic emotions.
Empathy	Appreciation of another's problems and feelings without experiencing the same emotional reaction.
Empirical	Greek *empeirikos*, experienced. Based upon observation or experience, and capable of being tested by observation or experiment.
Endophenotype	AKA intermediate phenotype. A *heritable* trait or characteristic that is not a direct symptom of the condition but is associated with that condition.
Epidemiologic Catchment Area (ECA) study	Epidemiologic Catchment Area (ECA) was a longitudinal study conducted from 1980 to 1985, which collected

data on the prevalence and incidence of mental disorders in New Haven, Baltimore, St. Louis, Durham and Los Angeles. A total of 20,861 patients were studied. The study provided the first definitive look at the state of mental health in the USA.

Erotomania
A delusional belief that another person, usually of a higher social status, is in love with them.

Ethnicity
The classification of a population that shares a common culture and national origin.

Executive functions
Higher-order cognitive functions involved in setting goals, planning, self-regulating and completing an intended task.

Expressed emotion
Negative communication by family members involving excessive criticism, emotional over-involvement and intrusiveness directed at a patient.

Extrapyramidal
Related to controlling and coordinating movement by the basal ganglia.

Faith
The relational aspects of religion. Among its many meanings are loyalty to a religion or religious community or its tenets, commitment to a relationship with God and belief in the existence of God.

Flat affect
Absent or almost absent affective expression.

Flight of ideas
Speech characterized by abrupt changes from topic to topic, generally with comprehensible associations.

fMRI
Functional MRI used to measure hemodynamic signals related to neural

	activity, by taking advantage of changes in the blood flow (and oxygenation) in such areas.
Gender	Perception of masculine or feminine, which is largely culturally determined, in contrast to the biological sex.
Gliosis	Proliferation of glia in damaged areas of the central nervous system ('scarring').
Grandiosity	Inflated self-estimation (worth, power, importance, knowledge, position), which can reach delusional proportions.
Gustatory	Latin *gustatio*, taste; pertaining to sense of taste.
Hallucination	False sensory perception in the absence of an external stimulus.
Heritability	Proportion of the observed variation in a particular phenotype that is attributable to the genotype.
Hyperprolactinemia	Increased levels of prolactin in the blood (normal: less than 20 ng/ml for women, and less than 15 ng/ml for men).
Hypochondria	False belief that one is suffering from a serious illness.
Hypofrontality	Reduction in prefrontal activity, measured by regional cerebral blood flow (rCBF) or PET; hypofrontality has been observed in schizophrenia.
Ideas of reference	Incorrect interpretations of innocuous incidents or belief that external events are of personal significance.
Illusion	Distortion of sensory perception in the presence of an external stimulus.
Incidence	Number of newly diagnosed cases during a specific time period.

Insight	Awareness and understanding of the origin and meaning of one's attitudes, feelings and behaviors and their effect on the person's environment (people and situations).
Labile, lability	Abnormal variability in affect with abrupt and unpredictable shifts.
Leukopenia	Decrease in total number of leukocytes (down to 4000–5000/mm³).
Lifetime prevalence	The number of individuals in the population who will develop the disorder at some point during their lifetime.
Linkage	Tendency for alleles at different loci to be inherited together. Thus, two 'linked' alleles are more likely to be inherited together. This observation is taken advantage of in linkage studies, in which co-segregation of the disease and genetic marker within families is examined.
Lobotomy	Outmoded surgical interruption of nerve tracts to and from the frontal lobe with the aim of treating intractable disorders such as schizophrenia and depression. The method was introduced by the Portuguese neurologist Egas Moniz in 1936, for which he was awarded the Nobel Prize.
Loose associations	Thinking characterized by tenuous connection between one thought (usually a sentence) and the next. When severe, speech becomes completely incomprehensible.
Magical thinking	Belief that one's thoughts, words or actions can result in outcome that defies normal laws of cause-and-effect.

Mannerisms	Goal-directed behaviors carried out in an odd or stilted fashion.
Morbid risk	The likelihood that an individual will develop a disease during a specific period or between specific ages.
MRI	Magnetic resonance imaging; see also fMRI.
Multifactorial	When a phenotype is determined by multiple genetic *and* non-genetic factors.
Myth	Greek *mythos*, a secret word or speech. Story or body of stories based on tradition or legend about the origins of the world, the causes of natural events and the origins of the society's customs and practices.
Negative symptoms	A cluster of symptoms characterized by diminution of mental function, frequently accompanied by motor symptoms (alogia, affective flattening, anhedonia, asociality, avolition and apathy and attentional impairment).
Neologism	Invention of word or the highly idiosyncratic use of a standard word ('my skull was completely fenestrated').
Neuroleptic	A compound that has both antipsychotic and extrapyramidal effects. The term was coined in 1952 by J. Delay, who introduced chlorpromazine to psychiatry.
Neuropil	Brain tissue that lies between the neurons.
Neutropenia	Decreased neutrophils in the peripheral blood. The absolute neutrophil count (ANC) defines neutropenia, derived by multiplying the percentage of bands and neutrophils on a differential by the

	total white blood cell count. An abnormal ANC is fewer than 1,500 cells per mm^3.
Nosology	Greek *nosos*, disease. The classification of diseases.
Olfaction	The sense of smell.
Open-ended question	A question that allows free-flowing responses (i.e. in their own words).
Orthostatic hypotension	Drop in systolic and diastolic pressures leading to postural symptoms (lightheadedness).
Overvalued idea	An unreasonable belief that is held with less than delusional intensity and is at odds with the community's cultural and religious beliefs.
P50	Brain-electrical responses to discrete stimuli, called event-related potentials (ERP), can be measured by EEG. The ERP waveform contains several components, including the latency period after a stimulus. Thus, P50 is an early component of the ERP, with '50' representing 50 milliseconds after the stimulus. P200 and P300 represent longer periods. These measurements have been used in schizophrenia research to study cognitive processes.
Paranoia	Irrational fear, suspicion or distrust of others that may reach delusional proportions.
Paraphrenia	Refers, in general, to late-onset schizophrenia (after age 45).
Parkinsonism	Having the characteristics of Parkinson's disease (resting tremor, rigidity, bradykinesia, postural instability and shuffling gait).

Penetrance	The extent to which the properties controlled by a gene are expressed. *Incomplete penetrance* is when less than 100% of the gene's properties are expressed in an individual.
Perception	The process of acquiring, interpreting and organizing sensory information from the environment or one's own body.
Perinatal	The period that includes fetal and neonatal periods, defined currently as from 20 weeks' gestation to 28 days after birth.
Perseveration	The persistence of verbal or motor response from a *previous* task occurring in the current task.
PET	Positron emission tomography (PET) is a method for imaging cerebral blood flow (presumed to reflect brain activity) by using radioactive tracers, which are injected into the bloodstream.
Phenomenology	Refers to the study of clinical phenomena, primarily signs and symptoms.
Point prevalence	The number of individuals in a population affected by a particular disease at a single point in time.
Polygenic	Phenotype caused by the interaction of multiple genes, each of which has a relatively small effect.
Polymorphism	Variations in the structure of the DNA sequences that permit genetic linkage analyses.
Positive symptoms	The productive symptoms seen in schizophrenia (delusions, hallucinations, thought disorder).
Posturing	The assumption of odd postures.

Poverty of *content* of speech	Speech is adequate or even excessive in amount but conveys little information because it is overinclusive, vague, concrete and repetitive.
Poverty of speech	Speech is characterized by brief and simple responses and little spontaneous speech; also called alogia.
Premorbid	Preceding the onset of illness.
Prevalence	Frequency of new and old (live) cases within a population at a given time point.
Primitive reflexes	AKA infantile responses. These are a group of reflex (motor) responses found during early development; most of these reflexes are inhibited during maturation, but can be 'released' in adulthood by cerebral damage. Examples of infantile responses that are later inhibited include sucking, startle, grasp, step and crawl.
Prognosis	Greek, *pro+gnosis*, foretelling. Predicting the probable course of disease.
Proprioception	Latin *proprius*, one's own. Awareness of the position of parts of the body in space in relation to one another.
Pruning	More properly *synaptic pruning*, which is normal elimination of synapses in the brain. The synapses and neurons most activated during growth are preserved.
Psychoeducation	Education (for patient and family) that serves the goals of treatment and rehabilitation; it includes information about the illness and its treatment, identifying signs of relapse, coping strategies and problem-solving skills.

Psychosis	Psychosis is a state characterized by loss of contact with reality, with a variety of manifestations – false beliefs (delusions), false perceptions (hallucinations), irrational thinking and behaviors.
QTc interval	QT interval represents the duration of ventricular depolarization and subsequent repolarization. QT interval prolongation is associated with cardiac arrhythmias. Because the QT interval varies with heart rate, the QT interval is 'normalized' into a heart-rate independent 'corrected' value, the QTc interval.
Race	Distinct human populations commonly distinguished on the basis of skin color, facial features, ancestry, genetics or national origin.
Recessive	Gene or trait that does not express in the presence of a dominant gene; two copies of the recessive gene are required for expression; indicated by lower-case letters (e.g. Aa).
Recovery	The absence of symptoms and return to premorbid level of functioning. Some definitions also include no further requirement for treatment and no longer being viewed as psychiatrically ill.
Relapse	It is generally understood to mean clinical worsening that requires active intervention, ranging from adjustment of APD dose to hospitalization.
Relativism	A view that humans understand and evaluate beliefs and behaviors in terms of a cultural context.

Religion	The belief in the supernatural, sacred or divine, and the moral codes, practices, values and institutions associated with such belief. Or we might say that religion is a belief in spiritual beings; but most understand religion to mean organized religion, for example Buddhism, Christianity, Hinduism, Islam and Judaism.
Restricted affect	Observable reduction in affective expression, not as severe as blunted affect.
Self-efficacy	The ability to cope with a situation – a concept that is important in the self-management of schizophrenia.
Sex	Male or female, identified on the basis of genetic and physical or biological characteristics.
Sialorrhea	Drooling or excessive salivation; the pooling of saliva beyond the margin of the lip.
Single-blind design	A type of (clinical) trial in which the subject does not know what treatment he or she is receiving, in order to minimize expectation.
Smooth-pursuit eye movements (SPEM)	Slow eye movements that function to maintain a slowly moving image on the fovea by matching eye velocity to target velocity.
Soft signs	Minor ('soft') neurological abnormalities in sensory and motor performance identified by clinical examination. 'Soft', as opposed to 'hard', reflects the absence of any obvious localized underlying neurological pathology.

Somatic	Perception of a physical experience localized within the body.
Somatosensory	Perception originating elsewhere in the body other than in the special sense organs (e.g. eyes).
SPECT	Single photon emission computed tomography (SPECT) is a method of brain scanning using radioactive dyes (that emit gamma rays), showing areas of increased metabolic activity. It is less specific than PET.
Spirituality	Often used interchangeably with religion, it may or may not include belief in supernatural beings and powers, but emphasizes experience at a personal level. Spirituality can mean a sense of connectedness or purpose, and that such experiences can facilitate personal development.
Stereognosis	The ability to recognize an object placed in the palm of the hand with eyes closed; disturbance in this ability (*asterognosis*) may indicate deficits in the contralateral sensory cortex.
Stereotypies	Non-purposeful and uniformly repetitive motions, such as tapping or rocking.
Stigma	Greek *stigma*, mark. A mark of disgrace, sign of moral blemish, stain or reproach.
Syndrome	Group or recognizable pattern of signs and symptoms or phenomena that indicate a particular trait or disease; the presence of one feature of the group alerts to the presence of the others.
Tangentiality	Thought disturbance in which thoughts/speech start off linearly, but

	quickly digress to unrelated areas without returning to the original point.
Tardive dyskinesia (TD)	Late-onset (tardive) abnormal movements characterized by non-rhythmic choreiform (jerky) or athetoid (slow, writhing) movements typically affecting the tongue, lips, jaw, fingers, toes and trunk. TD can be transient or permanent.
Therapeutic alliance	Collaborative relationship between patient and therapist.
Thought blocking	In mid-sentence the patient appears to have lost the train of thought.
Thought broadcasting	A sense that others can read one's thoughts.
Thought insertion	Belief or experience that outside forces or entities place thoughts into one's mind.
Titration	Stepwise increase or decrease in the dose of a medication.
Verbigeration	Frequent repetition of same word or phrase.
Volition	Commonly understood to mean the *will* towards action, choice or motivation. Lack of motivation (*avolition*) is seen in schizophrenia and classified as one of the negative symptoms.
Word salad	Speech is characterized by unconnected words or short, meaningless phrases.
Working memory	A type of memory *system* that involves the short-term retention and manipulation of information and integration of this transformed information into existing information (not to be confused with *short-term memory*, which is a component of working memory).

Helpful resources

Professional organizations

American Psychiatric Association (www.psychiatry.org)
A professional organization for psychiatry in the United States, and one of the largest psychiatric societies in the world.

International Early Psychosis Association (IEPA) (www.iepa.org.au)
A non-profit international network for those involved in the study and treatment of the early phases of mental-health disorders encompassing a trans-diagnostic approach.

National Institute of Mental Health (NIMH) (nih.gov)
The largest source of support for psychiatric research; also provides information for patients and families.

National Alliance for the Mentally Ill (NAMI) (www.nami.org)
An organization of families, consumers and professionals dedicated to the care of the mentally ill.

National Institute for Health and Care Excellence (UK) (www.nice.org.uk)
An excellent source for up-to-date practice guidelines and general information about the care of individuals with a variety of illnesses.

One Mind (onemind.org)
A leading brain-health nonprofit committed to mental-health advocacy.

Schizophrenia and Psychosis Action Alliance (sczaction.org)
A leading nonprofit organization advocating for brain health in individuals with serious mental illness.

Schizophrenia International Research Society (schizophreniaresearchsociety.org)
An international professional organization committed to promoting research in schizophrenia and related disorders.

Books

Cahalan, S. (2013). *Brain on fire: My month of madness.* Simon & Schuster.

D'Souza, D., Castle, D., & Murray, R. (2023). *Marijuana and madness* (3rd ed.). Cambridge University Press.

Duckworth, K. (2022). *You are not alone: The NAMI guide to navigating mental health – with advice from experts and wisdom from real people and families.* National Alliance on Mental Illness.

Freudenreich, O., Cather, C., & Stern, T. (2021). *Facing serious mental illness: A guide for patients and their families.* Massachusetts General Hospital Psychiatry Academy.

Fuller Torrey, E. (2019). *Surviving schizophrenia: A family manual* (7th ed.). HarperPerennial.

Insel, T. (2022). *Healing: Our path from mental illness to mental health.* Penguin Press.

Keshavan, M., & Eack, S. (2019). *Cognitive enhancement in schizophrenia and related disorders.* Cambridge University Press.

Lieberman, J. (2022). *Malady of the mind: Schizophrenia and the path to prevention.* Scribner.

Mueser, K. T., & Gingrich, S. (2006). *The complete family guide to schizophrenia: Helping your loved one get the most out of life.* Guilford Press.

Reddy, R., & Keshavan, M. (2015). *Understanding schizophrenia: A practical guide for patients, families, and health care professionals.* Praeger.

Tamminga, C., van Os, J., Reininghaus, U., & Ivleva, E. (2020). *Psychotic disorders: Comprehensive conceptualization and treatments.* Oxford University Press.

Practice guidelines

Australian Early Psychosis Guidelines. orygen.org.au

Keepers, G. A., Fochtmann, L. J., Anzia, J. M., Benjamin, S., Lyness, J. M., Mojtabai, R., Servis, M., Walaszek, A., Buckley, P., Lenzenweger, M. F., Young, A. S., Degenhardt, A., Hong, S. H., & (Systematic Review). (2020, September 1). The American psychiatric association practice guideline for the treatment of patients with schizophrenia. *American Journal of Psychiatry, 177*(9), 868–872.

National Institute of Clinical Excellence (NICE) guidelines. (2014). *CG178 psychosis and schizophrenia in adults.* nice.org.uk

Remington, G., Addington, D., Honer, W., Ismail, Z., Raedler, T., & Teehan, M. (2017, September). Guidelines for the pharmacotherapy of schizophrenia in adults. *Canadian Journal of Psychiatry. Revue Canadienne de Psychiatrie, 62*(9), 604–616.

Index

Note: Page numbers in *italics* indicate a figure and page numbers in **bold** indicate a table on the corresponding page.

A

Abilify (*see* aripiprazole)
accessory symptoms 146
affective blunting 21
agitation: management 132; in psychotic episode 73; treatment of 101
agranulocytosis, management **94**
akathisia: management **94**; in psychotic episode 73; and smoking 140
Alcoholics Anonymous (AA) 88
alcohol avoidance 109; and psychosis 40
algorithmic approach to diagnosis of schizophrenia/psychotic disorder 37–*38*
algorithms for susceptibility biomarkers 168
alogia 21
American Psychiatric Association 147
anger, assessment strategy 24
ANGUISH (consequences of stigma) 6
anhedonia 21
anorgasmia, management **94**
antianxiety agents, as aid in introduction of APDs 119
antipsychotic drugs (APDs) 65–67; advantages and disadvantages 66; atypical 66; avoidance 67; discontinuation by patient 68; long-acting depot 115–116; prescriptive characteristics 68–69; selection 68–**71**; titration 71; treatment duration 71; typical 66
antipsychotic drugs (APDs): general and range of severity 93–98; general principles 91–92; side effects 71
anxiety: in schizophrenia 22; as a side effects of APDs 180; treatment of 64, 81, 104, 182–183
aripiprazole **66, 69** (*see* Abilify)
asenapine **70** (*see* Saphris)
asociality 21
assessment: of schizophrenia 9–24; social determinants affecting 25–32
assertive community treatment (ACT) **79**, 86
attention deficit 22
auditory hallucinations **17**–18
automatic thoughts 81
avolition 21

B

behavior, violent, risk factors 131–132
behavioral disturbances 22

benzodiazepines: in agitation 73; for insomnia 73–74; for violence 132–133
biological factors 26–28, 32
biomarkers 167–168
bipolar I disorder 42; severe, with psychotic features 42
bipolar II disorder, severe with psychotic features 42
birth season **155**
Bleuler, Eugen 145–146
blurred vision, management of **94**
brain associated disturbances 157; imaging in diagnosis 40; progressive lesions 158; static lesions 158; structural abnormalities *159*; tissue reduction 157–158, *158*; brain network alterations 160
brexpiprazole **70** (*see* Rexulti)
Brief Psychiatric Rating Scale (BPRS) 99
brief psychotic disorder **43**
bromocriptine **96**

C
cannabis abuse **155**
cannabis-induced psychotic disorders **41**
Caplyta **71** (*see* lumateperone)
cardiological side effects of APDs **97**, 106,
cariprazine **70** (*see* Vraylar)
case management **79**, 86; mobile 88
catatonia **22**
chlorpromazine 65
chlorpromazine equivalents 71, **72–73**
circumstantiality 18
Clérambault's syndrome **16**
Clinical High Risk (CHR) 63
clinician: cultural competency 30; questions about illness 54; and religion 36
clozapine **66**, **69**, 106 (*see* Clozaril); 5-HT blocker 162; with aripiprazole 105; for depression in schizophrenia 138; metabolic syndrome **66**; side effects 96; for violence 132
Clozaril **69** (*see* clozapine)

cognitive abnormalities 22
cognitive behavioral therapy (CBT) 81; terms used in 81
cognitive deficits **22–23**
cognitive enhancement therapy (CET) 84
cognitive remediation 84
cognitive restructuring 81
cognitive therapy techniques 82
cognitive training 84–85
collaboration 91
communication 47–57
communities with high prevalence rates 150
compliance: and family 51; optimizing treatment with *104*; preventing relapse *125*; therapy 82
complications, treatment-related, management 91–98
computed tomography (CT) 157–158
confidentiality 51–52
consent 91
constipation, management **94**
Coordinated Specialty Care (CSC) 59–60
crisis intervention 88
cultural diversity 32
culture 29–30; and illness presentation 25
culture-bound psychotic disorder **44**

D
dantrolene **96**
decompensation: definition 121; management 123–125; measures to reverse 125, *125*; risk factors *122*
delusional disorder **43**
delusions: assessment 15–16; attitude to 13; BARRED **80–81**; common **15–16**; questions for diagnosis 16; uncovering 24
dependance/independence issues 51
depression: co-morbid *104*, 138, 141; in schizophrenia *42*, 138; severe, with psychotic features 41; and substance abuse 139
dermatoglyphics 179
developmental issues 164–165
developmental model *164*
diabetes 95, 106

Diagnostic and Statistical Manual of
  Mental Health 4th ed see DSM-IV
Diagnostic and Statistical Manual of
  Mental Disorders (DSM-5) 36, *38*
disorganized behaviour **44**, 161
disorganized speech **44**
dopamine excess theory *161*
dopamine hypothesis, revised 161
droperidol 132
drugs: addition of another
  104–105; changing 107; clinical
  trials 169; concentration in body
  102–103; illicit 6, 40, 109, 165;
  in development 169–170, **171**;
  dosage and smoking status 140;
  dose lowering 105; dose raising
  105; noncompliance, and relapse
  123; receptor responsivity 103
dry mouth see xerostomia,
  management of
DSM-IV 41, 147
DSM-IV-TR criteria for
  schizophrenia **44**
Duration of Untreated Psychosis
  (DUP) 60
dysphoria, treatment related 112
dystonia management **95**; and
  smoking 40

E
early intervention: design of
  61–62; opportunities for *60*; and
  prevention 62–63; service care
  pathway *61*
echolalia **22**
echopraxia **22**
ejaculatory dysfunction,
  management **95**
emotional disturbances 20
empathy, in assessment 10
employment, supported **79**, 87
endophenotypes 152–153, *153*
environmental factors 31, 154; in
  recovery 135
environmental risk factors **155**
Epidemiologic Catchment Area
  (ECA) study 181
erectile dysfunction, management **95**
erotomanic delusions **16**
etiological factors *152*
ethnicity and race 26, 28

executive functions, deficit **23**
expressed emotion (EE) 83

F
faith: beneficial 34; definition 33
family: language 52; hope,
  maintaining 52–53; intervention
  83, **79**; questions about illness 54;
  sessions 51–52; talking to 49–50;
  therapy 83; typical responses to
  illness 49
family interventions 83
Fanapt **71**
Federal Drug Administration (FDA)
  169
first-episode psychosis (FEP)
  patients 59
first-generation (APDs) **66**
flight of ideas **19**
fluphenazine **66**
folie à deux 43
Food and Drug Administration
  (FDA) 106
Freud, Sigmund 146
functional recovery 135

G
gamma-amino butyric acid
  (GABA) 162
gastrointestinal (liver enzyme
  elevation) side effects of APDs **96**
gender 27
gender differences **27**
gene-environment interaction 150,
  154–156
genes, search for 153
genetics 150–156
Geodon **69**
glucose metabolism abnormality,
  management **95**
glutamate 162
grandiose delusions **16**
gustatory hallucinations **18**

H
habit training 146
hallucinations 17–18; coping with
  80; observations in patients **17**;
  questions for diagnosis 16–17;
  uncovering **24**
haloperidol **66**, 132

Haslam, John 145
health belief model 111
Hecker, Ewald 145
heritability 151–*152*, 156
Hierarchical Taxonomy of
    Psychopathology (HiTOP) 147
histopathological studies 163
HOPE mnemonic 52–53
HOPES *31*
housing, supported 85, 87
humor, in assessment 10
hyperprolactinemia, management 95
hyperthermia, management 95
hypotension, orthostatic,
    management 96

I
illusions 17
iloperidone 71
I'M SCARED components 79
imagination, therapeutic 13
immigration 30–31
individualized psychotherapy *78*
insight 35; lack of 112
insomnia, management 73–74
INSPIRES approach 48
intensive case management (ICM) 79
International Classification of
    Diseases 146
International Pilot Study of
    Schizophrenia 25, *28*
interview, possibly psychotic
    persons 9–13

J
Jamaican immigrants, high
    schizophrenia rate 150

K
Kahlbaum, Karl 145
Kraepelin, Emil 145

L
language deficit 23
Latuda 70 (*see* lurasidone)
leukopenia, management 96
libido decrease, management 96
lifestyle 35
lipid abnormalities, management 96
liver enzyme elevation,
    management 96

location 31
long-acting depot antipsychotic
    agents (LAIs) 115–118
loose associations 19
lumateperone 71 (*see* Caplyta)
lurasidone 70 (*see* Latuda)

M
magnetic resonance imaging (MRI)
    studies 157–160
major depressive disorder 42
mannerisms 22
medical disorders, hallucinations
    in 17
memory deficit 23
mental status examination
    (MSE) 14
mesolimbic dopamine system 160
metabolic syndrome 66
Meyer, Adolf 146
mindfulness-based therapies 82
mood disorder with psychotic
    features 41
Morel, Benedict 145
motivational interviewing (MI) 82
motor coordination abnormalities 23

N
narcissism concept 146
Narcotics Anonymous (NA) 88
nature (genes) 150
negative symptoms 20–21;
    assessment 24; primary 20;
    secondary 20
neologism 19
neuroanatomical alterations
    157–160
neurobiology 157–166
neurochemical alterations 160–165
neurofeedback 168–169
neuroleptic malignant syndrome,
    management 96
neurological abnormalities 23
neuromodulation 168–169
neuronal connections, adolescent
    synapse pruning 164
neuronal density *164*
neuropathological evidence 163
neurophysiological alterations 163
neurotransmitter systems 162–163
neutropenia 185

non-adherence: assessment 110; causes 111; consequences 110; LEAP 112; management 112–113; management strategies 113; suspicion of 112
non-compliance *see* non-adherence
nurture (environment) 150

O
olanzapine **66**, 67, *68*; in agitation 73; dosage 105; glucose metabolism abnormality **95**; lipid abnormalities **96**; metabolic syndrome **66**; side effects **96**; and weight gain 105
olfactory hallucinations 17, **17–18**
Othello syndrome **16**

P
paranoia, assessment strategy **24**
paranoid delusions **15**
paraphrenia 146
parasuicide 129
parkinsonism: management **96**; and smoking 140
passivity delusions **16**
patient: questions about illness 49; talking about assessment 47–48; talking about treatment 49
patient health questionnaires (PHQ-9) 130
patient-related recovery factors 122
peer support 83
perception deficit 17
perinatal complications **155**
perseveration **19**
personal recovery 135
pharmacotherapy 77; *see also* treatment
Pinel, Phillipe 143
positive symptoms 20
positron emission tomography (PET) 160, 187
posturing **22**
poverty 31
prayer, helpful 35
precision psychiatry 170–172, *172*
prediction of outcome 55–56
prevalence 149; geographical variations 150; lifetime 149–150
primary psychotic disorder **41**

primitive reflexes, abnormalities 23
proactive approaches to nonadherence 111
prognostic factors 52
projection concept 146
psychiatric disorders, associated with psychosis 2
psychobiology 146
psychoeducation 77–78; principles 79–80
psychosis: due to medical condition 39–41; due to substance abuse 35; first-episode, drug treatment 67; imagining 13–14; major component assessment 14–18; relapse, drug treatment 67; religious themes in 33
psychosocial development and gender 27
psychosocial interventions 77
psychosocial stressors, effect on treatment response 102
psychotherapy 78
psychotic disorders **41**; interviewing patients 9
psychotic episode, common problems in 73–74

Q
Q-Tc prolongation, management **97**
questioning: manner of 12–13; patients 1–6
questions: how much and when 11–12; suicidal patient 11
quetiapine 67, **72** (*see* Seroquel); dosage **118**; and weight gain 105

R
reactive approaches to nonadherence 112
reactive psychosis **43**
recognition deficit **23**
recovery 85–86; factors influencing 135; in serious mental illness *136*; promotion 85–86; relations between factors influencing 136
referential thinking **16**
rehabilitation 86–87, 135–136
relapse 49; family therapy 83; impending, warning signs **124**; management 125–126; prediction

121–123; prevention 126; risk factors 122–123; warning symptoms 123
relativism 11
relaxation techniques **80**
religion: and clinician 35–36; definition 33; and psychiatry 36; and psychosis 34–35
religious delusions, assessment 34
religious experiences, normative and pathological 35
Research Domain Criteria (RDoC) framework 147
Rexulti **70** (*see* brexpiprazole)
risk evaluation and mitigation system (REMS) 106
Risperdal **69**
risperidone **69**, 73; dosage 103

S
Saphris **70** (*see* asenapine)
schemas 81
schizoaffective disorder **43**
schizophrenia: assessment 9–24; brain changes 165; characteristic symptoms **44**; co-morbid conditions 138–341; conceptual contributions **144**; consequences *3*; definition 1–2; development risk *151*; diagnostic steps 47–55; differential diagnosis **39**; etiological factors in *152*; heritability 151; history of 143–147; illness course 55; incidence 214; liability for 152; myths regarding 3, **4–6**; natural course 143; neurochemical 'imbalance' in *162*; outcome and course of 54–55, *56*; pathophysiological models of *165*; pathways 55; prevention 59–63; schizoaffective and Mood disorder exclusion 41–42; social withdrawal **45**; stigma 3; substance/medical condition **6**; transmission 151–152
schizophrenia spectrum disorders 152
schizophreniform disorder **43**
Schneider, Kurt 146
second-generation APDs (SGAs) 66
sedation, management **97**
seizures, management **97**
selective serotonin reuptake inhibitors (SSRIs) 138
sensory integration abnormalities 23
Seroquel **69** (*see* quetiapine)
serotonin 162
services research 172
shared psychotic disorder **43**
sialorrhea, management **97**
side effects 67–75
sleep evaluation clinic 74
smoking, cigarette, in schizophrenia 140
Smooth Pursuit Eye Movement (SPEM) dysfunction 152
social cognition deficits, treatment 84
social determinants of health (SDoH) 25, 154
social skills training (SST) 85
soft signs 23
somatic delusions **16**
somatosensory hallucinations **18**
spirituality, description 33
stereotypies **22**
stress reduction 102; and relapse 123; role of, in family 47; sources for migrants 30; vulnerability to 152
substance abuse 40–42, 88; and relapse 123; in schizophrenia 139, 141
Substance Abuse and Mental Health Services Administration (SAMHSA) 130
substance-induced psychotic disorder 50
suicide, risk factors 129–133
supernatural, belief in 33
supported employment 87
symptoms: management 86; pharmacological management 65–74
synapse, decreased density 164
syndromal recovery 135

T
tachycardia, management **97**
tangentiality **19**

tardive dyskinesia (TD)
    management 97
TEACH components 79
therapeutic alliance 47, 51
thiothixene 66
thought blocking 19
thought broadcasting 16
thought disorder, uncovering *20*
thought disturbance 18, *20*;
    observations in patients 21;
    questions for diagnosis 26
thought insertion 16
treatment: approaches to 102;
    continuous services 136;
    improved outcome 25; inadequate
    response, causes 101–103; non-
    adherence 82, 91, 102; response
    continuum *100*; suboptimal
    response 103–106, *104*; *see also*
    pharmacotherapy; side effects
treatment-resistant schizophrenia
    (TRS) 99, 106
treatment response and resistance
    in psychosis (TRRP) 99

V
verbigeration 19
violence management 131;
    persistent 131; reduction
    programs 132; transient 132
vision, blurred, management 94
visual hallucinations 17–18
Vraylar 70 (*see* cariprazine)
vulnerability markers 152

W
weight gain, management 98
word salad 19
World Health Organization (WHO)
    25, 146

X
xerostomia, management of 94

Z
ziprasidone 66, 67, 69; in
    agitation 73
Zydis 68 (*see* Zyprexa)
Zyprexa 68 (*see* Zydis)

For Product Safety Concerns and Information please contact our EU
representative GPSR@taylorandfrancis.com
Taylor & Francis Verlag GmbH, Kaufingerstraße 24, 80331 München, Germany